101 Tips

FOR THE PARENTS OF

BOYS WITH AUTISM

101 Tips

FOR THE PARENTS OF

BOYS WITH AUTISM

The Most Crucial Things You Need to Know About
Diagnosis, Doctors, Schools, Taxes, Vaccinations,
Babysitters, Treatment, Food, Self-Care, and More

Ken Siri

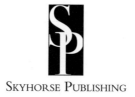

Skyhorse Publishing

Skyhorse Publishing books may be purchased in bulk at special discounts for sales promotion, corporate gifts, fund-raising, or educational purposes. Special editions can also be created to specifications. For details, contact the Special Sales Department, Skyhorse Publishing, 307 West 36th Street, 11th Floor, New York, NY 10018 or info@skyhorsepublishing.com.

Skyhorse® and Skyhorse Publishing® are registered trademarks of Skyhorse Publishing, Inc.®, a Delaware corporation.

Visit our website at www.skyhorsepublishing.com.

10 9 8 7 6 5 4 3

Library of Congress Cataloging-in-Publication Data is available on file.

ISBN: 978-1-62914-507-5
Ebook ISBN: 978-1-62914-841-0

Printed in China

WARNING: The information contained herein is for informational purposes only. Neither the editor, nor the publisher, nor any other person or entity can take any medical or legal responsibility of having the information contained within *101 Tips for the Parents of Boys with Autism* considered as a prescription for any person. Every child is different and parents need to consult with their own doctors, therapists, lawyers, financial advisors, or other professional to determine what is best for them and their child. Failure to do so can have disastrous consequences.

For my mother and father, who made all possible,
and
For all the parents out there working to improve the
lives of their kids.

Contents

Introduction

Things in themselves are always neutral, it is our perception which makes them appear positive or negative.

—Epictetus

I wrote this book to accomplish two missions, one, to educate myself on how best to manage the challenging life of a sole custody dad of a boy with autism, and second, to share what I learn and provide a short cut for those who follow.

Throughout the book I will comment on the Tips presented, which of course means that my experiences will guide my views. To that, I will share a bit of my background so you will understand these views.

I am a single, sole custody dad (for the last eight years) and caregiver for my son Alex, who is now sixteen years old. Alex and I live in Manhattan in a one-bedroom apartment. I used to work on Wall Street before I took full custody of Alex, but then transformed my life when he came to live with me in 2008. Since then I have started my own business, written books, spoken at conferences, become a board member for both the National Autism Association, New York Metro Chapter and The Atlas Foundation for Autism, and most importantly, positively shaped Alex's development.

Alex is presently non-verbal, communicating primarily with an iPad, has had autoimmune issues (ulcerative colitis), behavioral issues, and sensory issues. Alex currently attends public school in Manhattan, and previously attended a private autism school in Manhattan. He is improving physically, emotionally and mentally thanks to many of the tips herein.

Before we begin, I would like to share a couple of points that I have learned on this journey. First is to take ownership of all aspects of treatment, education, therapy, and organization and view yourself as a CEO. I am the CEO of Team Alex. To do this you will need to speak out and be prepared to fight for the rights of your child. The "squeaky wheel gets oiled" may not be fair, but that is the way to handle the many bureaucratic organizations and mindsets you will encounter.

Secondly is that to have the desired impact on your child and accept and acclimate to a life that one cannot be prepared for you will experience stress. Stress unimagined by those not in our autism universe. How much stress? There was a study done (several actually) where parents of children with autism were stress tested and compared to

Introduction

various professions—the closest equivalent, combat soldier. Not just a soldier mind you, but one in combat. Basically we autism parents are under fire 24/7. Because of this I will dwell significantly on Self-Care and some of the best strategies, ideas, and thoughts that have helped me and the many amazing parents I have met on my journey.

As those of us who are connected to this community know, no two kids on the spectrum are the same in behaviors, challenges, or talents. To that I have included Tips from other friends in the autism community to round out or cover areas missing in my experiences with Alex. In addition, these folks have provided some really great advice that just needs to be shared, so I do.

Finally, many parents are either going through or have gone through what you are feeling right now. I hope this book will educate, aid, and most importantly remind you that you are not alone and that there is help out there. Let us begin.

—Ken Siri
New York, NY
January 2015

Author's Note

This book seeks to provide helpful tips, general information, and strategies to help families master autism. This book is not intended to provide specific medical advice; all therapies and treatments discussed are for informational purposes only. All medical treatments have the potential for harmful side effects so seek the advice of your doctor before beginning any biomedical treatments for your child.

Autism is a spectrum, and all children with autism are different. What works for one child may not work for another. For this reason, some of these Tips may appear contradictory. As a parent, your first job is to observe your child and learn to use your intuition, so you can develop the sense, which will guide you to the most helpful advice. Also, these are Tips, not rules; try them out and adopt what works for you and your child.

I have grouped the Tips for easy future reference and there is an Index at the end of the book to facilitate finding Tips by Keyword. In addition, I have highlighted KEY TIPS that have been the most useful to Alex and I, and that I believe most in the community can all benefit from. If you try anything, try the KEY TIPS.

Some Tips have come from other parents and caregivers, and I have kept the voice of the various contributors. In doing so, I realize that different terminology is used when describing children with autism (child with autism, autistic child, child on the spectrum, aspie, child with Asperger's, high-functioning, more-able, etc.). Just remember the saying, "If you've seen one child with autism, you've seen one child with autism."

Chapter 1

Diet

diet

noun

1. the kinds of food that a person, animal, or community habitually
    eats: *a vegetarian diet* | *a specialist in diet.*
    *   a regular occupation or series of activities in which one
        participates: *a healthy diet of classical music.*
2. a special course of food to which one restricts oneself, either to
    lose weight or for medical reasons: *I'm going on a diet.*

The Gut/Brain Connection

Before getting into the Tips for dietary interventions, I
believe it important to state the why behind taking on
the challenge in the first place. Of course, all of us could
benefit from a cleaner, healthier diet. But more specific
to the autism population is the gut/brain connection.
Recently, research has been able to shed light on the
importance of this connection and how our western
diet and toxins may be responsible for alarming increases
in various autoimmune and brain related conditions.
The following is a piece I wrote which will help
answer the "why" behind the importance of Dietary
Interventions.

Autism, a punch to the gut?

Autism, Dementia and Gastrointestinal Issues

At the beginning of this month (December 2013) there were a couple of studies that came out which garnered some modest press. The first was "Dementia Epidemic Looms with 135 million Sufferers Expected by 2050." This particular headline was on Fox, but was similarly reported by multiple outlets (see 12/5/13 FoxNews.com).

The story highlighted the exponential growth expected in dementia, highlighted by Alzheimer's, going from 44 million to 135 million by 2050. Alzheimer's Disease International (ADI) said the study showed a 17% increase over two years, which when extrapolated forward gives the 135 million in 2050 figure. This growth rate is significantly higher than the world population growth of about 1.2% (US Census Bureau). More telling, the world population growth will be cut in half between now and 2050 to .6% (US Census again). The ADI called it a "global epidemic" which is only going to get worse. The current global cost of care for dementia is more than $600 billion, equal to about 1.0 percent. At 2050 we are talking about 3% of the global population having dementia given the estimates above, which will become a serious drag on global growth.

Now where have we come across numbers similar to this before? A subset of the population that is growing significantly faster than the population as a whole. A subset that should remain constant in percentage terms if it is genetic. And, a subset that seems to be growing along with another subset, or subsets actually. Yes, the autism and dementia growth rates are very similar. Possibly a coincidence. Possibly not. When you figure in the increasing rates of autoimmune conditions (which are also similar) and see that all seem to increase exponentially from the same base, the possibility of coincidence diminishes.

I find it interesting that we are not hearing about better diagnosis in terms of dementia, or autoimmune conditions, only in autism. SO what could be causing this?

WELL, a few days later, a second study, reported in multiple outlets, indicated that "autism may be linked to gastrointestinal issues" according to a study from Caltech (12/7/13).

The study evidenced that behaviors associated with autism are "influenced from gastrointestinal

(GI) issues, and could be treated with probiotic therapy." Researchers utilized a particular "good" human bacteria in a mouse model to treat induced GI & autism issues, what resulted was a decrease in GI troubles and autism-like symptoms. This led the scientists to theorize that behavioral issues on the autism spectrum may be caused by GI issues and can be treated by healing the gut.

The study also pointed out how "leaky gut," the induced GI condition, has also become a target of researchers in Parkinson's, multiple sclerosis and Alzheimer's; as other studies have tied these conditions to GI disease. What Caltech scientists conclude is "this suggests that GI problems could contribute to particular symptoms in neurodevelopmental disorders."

The specific connections investigated between autism and GI were: chronic constipation, diarrhea, reflux, IBD (Inflammatory Bowel Disease) in GI and; defects in social interaction, communication and repetitive behaviors in autism.

IT seems from all this that the increases in the neuro & autoimmune conditions may be linked by GI. Long thought to reside in the brain, perhaps all the trouble, or the cause of these conditions lies in the stomach/GI tract. If so, this would also lead one to believe the hypothesis that something, other than better diagnosis, is causing the exponential increase in these conditions. This brings us back to the heavy use of antibiotics, pesticides, drugs and other chemicals in our food supply, bodies and environment.

The HOPE is that this information will lead to more research and focus on the gut's impact on autism, dementia and all the above. The exciting implications of this, according to the researchers, is that the gut is far easier to study and address than the brain and potentially more impactful, as the mice in the study became more communicative and less anxious with treatment (particular probiotics). Stay tuned.

PS: As mentioned in previous articles, my son has had serious GI issues, including painful reflux and ulcerative colitis. Test results (scopes) of his GI tract led more than one doctor to date the beginning of his GI trouble to the approximate beginning of his autism regression (without knowing that he regressed). Treatments for GI issues have significantly benefited Alex and though still non-verbal, his behaviors, control and vocalizations have improved over the last two years of treatment (again for GI).

Starting a Diet

So, changing your child's diet is one of the most significant things you can do to impact your child's health. The Gluten-Free/ Casein-Free (GF/CF) diet is the most popular; we suggest removal of soy as well, as soy has properties similar to casein. Beyond this, the Specific Carbohydrate (SCD) Diet has been effective for those children who did not respond sufficiently to GF/CF.

I know that in the case of my son, Alex, the SCD diet has worked wonders. Alex, besides being autistic, also has ulcerative colitis (UC). The UC was quite severe and still requires potent medications, but he is healing at a tremendous pace and recently we were able to remove some meds (which is rare given the severity of where Alex's colitis was at when diagnosed). This is a key reason his gastrointestinal (GI) doctors credit the SCD diet for his progress.

~

Most pros think you should give the diet a good six months. Personally, I am always learning about new alternatives, and I feel that six months may be a bit short, given that it will likely take you months just to clean up the diet. It's best to adopt the diet as a family and look to make constant improvements to it over time; you'll all feel and perform better in the long run. As a rule of thumb, we typically have a protein item and three vegetables for a dinner, protein and vegetables and fruits for lunch. Breakfast is bacon and eggs for Alex (SCD legal) and fruit, or occasionally a nut based granola with almond or coconut milk.

~

If you begin to suspect a particular food item might be impacting behavior, test. Give your son two weeks away from the item and observe the results. It will be another clue for your medical team. Don't forget to remind folks at school about this, and other food restrictions.

Organizing a Diet

Keep a diary—this will turn out to be an important tool and should not be overlooked. Get a spiral pad or notebook and list each food your child eats on the left side of the page. On the right side of the page, list any changes you observe. Make a note of things like aggression, crying, whining, red ears, itchiness, bowel movements, stimming, tantrums, or sleep problems. Go high tech with this and create an excel workbook that is easy to update and keep track of dietary changes and their impact in a more visual way.

To this, I am offering my spreadsheet (in Excel) via the Skyhorse website. You can download it for free from www. skyhorsepublishing.com/book/?GCOI=60239108168770&

This spreadsheet has many uses, including dietary tracking, supplement tracking, and just getting organized.

Removal Strategies

Begin by removing all dairy products from the diet, and within a week or two, all gluten. Using sugars, rice, potatoes, and other starchy foods to achieve this transition may be necessary, but keep in mind that they will probably need to be reduced or even removed later on.

Consider removing soy and corn at the same time gluten is removed. Many parents have given up on the gluten-free diet because they saw no change or a regression in their children, after having substituted soy for milk or corn for gluten. These two foods are almost universally problematic when starting the diet. They can always be added back later on a trial basis.

The reason is that though soy in some cases can be a good substitute for milk, it does have some casein-like properties, which make it a candidate for removal after gluten. Best to avoid from the get-go. I suggest almond or coconut-based milk substitutes. They taste great and actually have higher levels of calcium and vitamin D.

~

Keep in mind that "nondairy" does not mean milk-free. It is a term the dairy industry invented to indicate less than 0.5

percent milk by weight, which could mean fully as much casein as whole milk.

~

When beginning to remove casein and then gluten (and perhaps other foods), phase out the products instead of the cold-turkey approach. First, it will make things easier to take for you and your child, and second, it gives you time to learn the various sources of these products in your diet. You'll be surprised and perhaps shocked at the extent of their use in the Western diet. To this end you need to eliminate not only gluten and casein but also any artificial ingredients and sugars. Focus on eating organic and local.

~

For some children, it might be necessary to simultaneously remove other foods, especially soy, corn, and even rice. Some children will require the elimination of all complex carbohydrates and others will need to reduce oxalates.

Picky Eaters

Don't force picky eaters to eat. Just prepare the healthy foods and serve. Give it a day or two while keeping them hydrated. Most kids will begin to try what is in front of them as soon as they grow hungry. For those who do not, a strategic retreat may be in order, but give it those couple of days first. If it's no go, fall back, look for more alternatives, and try again a week later. If after a few attempts you are having no luck, consult a nutritionist, and, other parents who have had success.

In our case, Alex would hold out to eat certain portions of his meal, then signal for more of what he wanted (meaning what he had finished already). By not giving in (or providing seconds of the preferred item) I was able to get him to try virtually any vegetable and food, and over time all resistance fell. On occasion he will try and hold out for a favored item (say hot dogs—SCD legal of course) over more vegetables, but he knows I am serious about skipping meals if necessary so he no longer tests me, much. Additionally, it is common to see crankiness, regression, or withdrawal symptoms during these first few days. Stay the course, and let your child know that you mean business.

~

"Fussy eating is a common problem. In some cases the child might be fixated on a detail that identifies a certain food. Hilde De Clercq found that one child only ate Chiquita bananas because he fixated on the labels. Other fruit such as apples and oranges were readily accepted when Chiquita labels were put on them. Try putting different but similar foods in the cereal box or another package of a favorite food. Another mother had success by putting a homemade hamburger with a wheat-free bun in a McDonald's package."

—Temple Grandin, PhD, author of *Thinking in Pictures and The Way I See It*; www.autism.com/ind_teaching_tips.asp

Tightening up a Diet

Depending on your child's sensitivity, you may need to get extreme in removing the products; if so, don't forget products like soaps, shampoos, and such. Alex used to put bubbles from his bath into his mouth. The problem: the soap contained casein, along with undesirable chemicals. Switch to a clean natural product, such as those by California Baby, to close this potential hole in the diet.

～

Put your son on an organic diet, and remove additives, preservatives, colorings, processed carbs, and sugars (and don't forget juice, which is usually mostly water and high fructose corn syrup). Instead, utilize complex carbs (slower absorption) and healthful proteins, then observe. This will provide clues on which diet to follow, and how strict implementation will need to be. Share these clues with your nutritionist and medical team for advice on what diets/treatments may work best.

～

Most cheese substitutes contain some form of casein. It can even be found in tuna fish and other canned foods. Many wheat-free cereals contain malt (from barley) and thus are not gluten-free. Chewing gum, stickers, Play-Doh—all of these can be sources of gluten and casein. In short, you need to be a detective and investigate everything that goes into your child's mouth. Remember that, especially with small children, nonfood items often end up there too. Just a trace can make a world of difference in your results.

Additionally, you might have heard recently of a study where researchers tested dozens of products labeled gluten-free, and found that 70 percent of them failed the test. What to do? Move away from all processed foods. Use "gluten/casein-free" processed products only as a stepping-stone to a cleaner diet. There are also many alternatives to processed items; for instance, dried fruit chips (Made in Nature, Bare Fruit Snacks) which we have successfully used.

~

Go fish. To eliminate the chance of ingesting toxins via food, avoid toxic fish, especially those that are the larger, longer-living species such as swordfish, which wind up absorbing more of the mercury and other toxins in the ocean. Others in the group include tilefish, marlin, and shark. Check out the following site from the Natural

Resources Defense Council for a more detailed list of fish with the most, and least mercury: www.nrdc.org/health/effects/mercury/guide.asp.

~

Use only Himalayan salt or sea salt. Himalayan in particular is the most clean, as the oceans contain chemicals including lead and mercury. Common refined table salt contains aluminum. Yes, aluminum. It is used to cut the salt and keep it from sticking. Needless to say, this is quite unhealthy, and it's important to know that aluminum enhances the toxicity of other toxins.

Offsetting Dietary Deficiencies

Getting Enough Calcium with the GF/CF Diet:

- Green vegetables such as kale, collards, and bok choy are excellent sources of calcium, with the added benefit of being low in oxalates (spinach, though high in calcium, should be avoided if oxalates are a problem).
- Certain fish, like salmon and perch, are also good sources of calcium, but take care to buy fish that is not high in mercury or other environmental toxins (focus on smaller, preferably non-farmed fish).
- A mere tablespoon of molasses contains 172 mg of calcium (as well as iron), so if yeast is not a big problem, it is a good choice for sweetening baked goods.

- Some nuts, beans, and seeds (like sesame seeds) are rich in calcium, but they should be ground for best absorption. Also note that almond milk has a higher concentration of calcium than cow's milk.

- Finally, if a child will not eat enough nondairy sources of calcium, there are many good supplements available. Because vitamin D is required to properly absorb calcium, a good supplement program will contain both. And with vitamin D, especially for those of us in northern latitudes with long winters, be sure to use a high IU count; experts advise upwards of 2,000. This is one of those core supplements that most of us should be on. Several studies have shown that kids on the spectrum are frequently deficient in this important vitamin.

~

Remember the prime source of vitamin D (which stimulates the production and use of calcium in the body) is the sun. Get enough sunlight on your child each day, about fifteen minutes will do, and skip the sunblock during this time. Worried about the rays? Take your fifteen minutes in the early morning or late day when the sun is "weaker."

Getting Help

Consider seeing a nutritionist or dietitian trained in the implementation of diets that have been successful for some people with ASD. The Autism Research Institute (ARI) maintains a list on their website (www.autism.com) of professionals who have attended their nutrition seminars.

~

Some of the most popular autism-diet groups include:

- Gluten-Free/Casein-Free Diet (GF/CF): www. yahoogroups.com/group/gfcfkids
- The Specific Carbohydrate Diet (SCD): www. yahoogroups.com/group/pecanbread
- The Low Oxalate Diet (LOD): www.yahoogroups. com/group/Trying_Low_Oxalates
- The Feingold Diet: www.yahoogroups.com/group/ Feingold-Program4us
- The Body Ecology Diet: www.bedrokcommunity.org

~

Get support: Compile a few articles on diet that you can give family members, teachers, and other caregivers. Tell them what you are doing, and why. Ask for their support, especially school staff, as they will have to enforce the diet in your absence. In our case, Alex had a few meltdowns/tantrums at schools he was new to. It turned out they had let him get hold of "illegal" items. Once I tied the behaviors to these items, staff became more diligent on keeping to his diet.

~

KEY TIP

I've mentioned this already, but please try the SCD diet, especially if your child has GI difficulties. It is one of the key variables in Alex's improvement and has helped me as well. To get started, read *Breaking the Vicious Cycle* by Elaine Gottschall and familiarize yourself with the legal/illegal list on the following website (www. breakingtheviciouscycle.info/home/). From here you will be led to menu changes, suggested recipes, and other helpful information.

~

Finally, while it might be challenging to have your entire family follow this dietary path, the benefits of introducing everyone to more pure, whole foods should be obvious. Just try and make changes in small batches, as too many adjustments at once are difficult to process, track, and keep. Slow and steady wins this race.

Chapter 2

Self-Care (for parents and caregivers)

The world is changed by your example, not your opinion.

—*Paulo Coelho*

Do Not Skip This Chapter!

Self-Care is frequently the most neglected part of caring for children with autism, especially those with significant needs. Whether it be time constraints, motivation, tiredness, or guilt, I find parents (and frequently caregivers) all too often do not take proper care of themselves. In this I include fitness, mental health, socializing with peers, and sleep. How many reading this place all these items on the back burner? Why? How can you care for your child long-term if you are not fit and healthy? If you have young children now, what about when they are larger than you? Are you worried about their future? How will you help them if you don't care for yourself now?

Think about your last flight. You know, the part that nobody pays attention to. "In event of an emergency, oxygen bags will drop from the ceiling, affix yours before putting on your child's." Why do they say this? Because you will be unable to help them if you are unable to function yourself. Heed this and practice some Self-Care. It's not just for you. It's for your child too.

Fitness

Run! No, not away from your concerns, but as a way to deal with them. You need exercise to keep fit for parenting, and nothing is easier, cheaper, or more fun than running. Running is also a bona fide stress reliever and provides an opportunity for your mind to organize its thoughts. Join a local running club or organization. Here in New York City we are blessed with the New York Road Runners, but there are many similar organizations around the country and if one is not near, you can start one.

When you get rolling with the running, drop the iPod and listen to yourself think. I also suggest you run with your son. What could be better? Get him involved, it can provide the same exercise, stress relief, and mental calming for him.

Reading

It may seem strange to include a reminder to read, in a book, but the fact is way too many folks just do not read enough. Statistics vary, but something like 50 percent of all books purchased are not read! Reading has so many benefits; for our purposes here, it is a calming activity and a great way to finish the day. Much better than TV, which does not promote sleep or active dreaming as reading can.

One great way to end the day is to read in a supine position on the floor with your legs up the wall. This helps stretch out your back, hamstrings, calves, and glutes, all of which need it after sitting all or much of the day. Your son can get into the act as well.

Speaking of TV, reading more can lead to less TV, which is good. Sorry TV, but facts are facts. Here is one example— by the age of sixty, the average American has spent fifteen years watching TV. Years! Think of that. What could you do with a spare fifteen years in life? I try to keep TV to a minimum with my reading/TV ratio. I want to read at least 2/1 or two hours reading per every hour of TV. What's your ratio? Later, you can begin to think of this ratio in regards to other activities, so what is your ratio of fitness activities/ TV? Thinking like this can motivate one to make the incremental adjustments over time that lead to significant change. Small changes lead to big benefits.

Counseling and Support Groups

Parent support groups can be an amazing resource. Not only can they provide support as you raise your child with autism, but they can also offer a place to find out information regarding treatments other parents have tried, tips from other parents about traveling or community outings, after-school activities, and much more. Other parents know what you are going through; they are full of information about their own experiences, and are usually more than willing to share and help another parent out.

The following Tips are by Lauren Tobing-Puente, PhD, from the chapter on "Parent Support" in *Cutting-Edge Therapies for Autism*.

- Individual counseling with a mental-health clinician allows opportunities for focusing on parents' own experiences and developing coping strategies that can help them manage their parenting stress and any symptoms of psychological distress. Here, they can specifically address their struggles in order to become more effective in their parenting roles and feel increased contentment overall.
- Marriage counseling with a mental-health clinician who has a background in families of children with ASDs is often helpful for addressing issues within the marriage. Support for the siblings of children with ASDs is also important for addressing the impact on the entire family.
- Parents should be as much the focus in treatment as the children themselves, as their well-being is critical to their ability to be a part of their children's therapy. The optimal functioning of the parents is essential if the treatment strategies are to be successfully implemented.
- Education regarding what is known about the cause(s) of ASDs is often crucial for parents who experience guilt

and self-blame. Listening to others who have had similar experiences helps parents feel a sense of community, contrasting their experience of isolation from others.

• Parent support groups, often led by a mental-health clinician, are provided regularly by many schools and local organizations. Such groups provide opportunities for parents to share their experiences, discuss ways of helping their children (e.g., by sharing information on treatment protocols and behavioral strategies), and caring for themselves. With the guidance of mental-health clinicians, parents can receive education about the latest research on ASDs and treatment and strategies that can help their children and themselves.

• Message boards and listservs for parents of children with ASDs have become very popular in recent years. The benefits of message boards and listservs include their convenience and accessibility, without the challenges of scheduling face-to-face support groups. This can be especially helpful for parents who live in remote areas. However, online technology does not afford the personal contact of support groups or provide the same opportunity to develop true relationships with other parents. Without consistent moderation by a clinician, it is difficult to ensure that the content is appropriate and factual.

~

A support system is crucial—and not just a family-and-friends system, but a group of people familiar with autism who might be able to help you out with the intricacies of the condition. Here in NYC I started an informal group of parents and caregivers that meet out socially once per month at my favorite restaurant, Calle Ocho. It's great fun, and perfect for sharing information and networking. Start one yourself.

Employment

In some cases, one or both parents may need to change or adjust their career plans to accommodate the care of a special needs child. As a single parent, the challenge can be daunting. Many are forced to work from home or go into business for themselves in order to provide the flexibility required to properly care for their child. I had to do this myself. Though it may be, initially, overwhelming and stressful, many parents have remade themselves successfully and found a greater satisfaction in building their own business. These are not really tips, but below are some benefits you can look forward to with the change.

- You control your own time—much time is wasted in a traditional job; working for yourself will make you more efficient and effective. You'll only do what is necessary to complete a task/job versus the office politics and endless meetings that provide no value and waste your time in a traditional setting. You'll get paid for what you can deliver, not how much time you spend at a desk. This is time which *you* lose that you can put to better use.

- You lose security in the traditional sense, but let's face it: a traditional job gives the illusion of security for a paycheck.

- Being your own boss means not having to beg someone else for money or a raise or wait to be noticed. You also do not have to deal with anyone you find negative or unsavory.

- Socially you'll be free. Most folks only socialize with those they work with, which means you don't typically have access to those with alternative mindsets and experiences, which is something required for growth and long-term mental health.

- When you work for someone else, notice how many folks complain about this or that on the job. Negativity abounds, because deep down, you do not want to serve someone else. Working for yourself or independently means you have no time for negative whining, only for getting things done.

KEY TIP

I am often asked "How do you do so much?" after I describe to folks what life is like for a single parent of a child with special needs. And yes, I do quite a bit, from being Alex's dad and sole caregiver, to running a business, writing, being involved in a film project and on the board of two autism organizations. I also did a couple of triathlons last year (including one Ironman) and multiple running races. How do I do so much? The key is stress management. Stress management incorporates several factors that I discuss in this book, but the absolute KEY factor is meditation. Not only can meditation help you accomplish more with less stress, but it also has other beneficial side effects. Here are some from recent research I came across. Later in the book I will discuss how you can set up and incorporate your own practice.

Meditation

- **More flexibility.** The more you meditate the faster your amygdala (a region shown in research to perform a primary role in the processing of memory, decision-making, and emotional reactions) can recover from stress and trauma. According to research published in *Frontiers in Human Neuroscience* in February 2012, "meditation can alter the geometry of the brain's surface. . . . There was a study done at the University of California in Los Angeles involving 50 meditators and 50 controls that addressed a possible link between meditation and cortical gyrification (which is the pattern and degree of cortical folding that allows the brain to process faster). . . . This study showed a positive correlation between the amount of gyrification in parts of the brain and the number of years of meditation for people, especially long-term meditators, compared to non-meditators . . . this increased gyrification may reflect an integration of cognitive processes when meditating, since meditators are known to be introspective and contemplative, using certain portions of the brain in the process of meditation."

- **More gray matter.** Just three months of meditation can create more gray matter in areas of the brain impacting self-awareness and compassion. Research published in the May 2013 edition of *Psychology Today* explains, "how the brain functions better with meditation, and the positive effects it has on the brain, the longer you meditate." The research shows "how the brain can be molded by meditation . . . specifically, the connection to our fear center and our ego center wither away—by meditating on a regular basis." This "molding" weakens the negative neural pathways associated with our feelings of anxiety and depression, which gives a chance for better (positive) neural pathways to be formed.

- **Less stress, fewer distractions, and more focus.** Meditation can quiet your overactive thinking, which can fill your mind with worries and distractions.

Meditation helps prevent your mind from wandering so you can stay focused on the task at hand. Meditation also blocks stress and protects your brain from stress-related damage to attention and memory. Researchers have found that those who practice meditation can adjust their brains waves better. They can screen out distractions and increase productivity faster than those who do not meditate. Less distraction gives room for the brain to integrate new information.

Mindfulness

"As a parent, you did not choose to have a boy with autism. However, you can choose how you are going to react and what you are going to do about it. The first step is to acknowledge the emotions you are feeling. Realize that all parents go through these emotions—they are real and unavoidable. These emotions have been likened to the five stages of grief that a person goes through when faced with the death of a loved one. In this case, your son is still here, but what you are mourning is the loss of your expectations, of everything you had hoped and dreamed for with the birth of your son. The second step is learning all you can to help your child recover or reach his full potential."

—Chantal Sicile-Kira, author of *Autism Spectrum Disorders*

CHAPTER 3

Biomedical

"Do the difficult things while they are easy and do the great things while they are small. A journey of a thousand miles must begin with a single step."

—Lao Tzu

Where to Begin?

For many parents, working through the various biomedical treatments and associated diets are the most challenging components of autism. It's easy to become overwhelmed with so much information. It's best to focus on one day and one treatment at a time, and remember—no matter how difficult the day, keep on breathing, because tomorrow is another day. The sun will rise, and who knows what Providence will bring.

~

Before starting down this road, remember that most recoveries and improvements have taken considerable time. In many cases your child has been "sick" for a while, and there is no quick fix. Think of biomedical therapy as a marathon that will take considerable time and perseverance, so you need to pace yourself. And, most important, a marathon is much more mental than physical; mental strength is the key. There is no magic bullet. Likewise, stay away from anyone offering a "cure," or anyone who professes that his or her method will work for everyone with an ASD.

Getting Going and Staying Motivated

When beginning biomedical therapies, it's best not to begin everything at once. Try to phase things in over the course of weeks and months so that you can determine what might and might not be working. If you start too much at once, you will not know what is working or what could be causing problems.

~

Look for the trend. During the course of biomedical treatments, you will see some progression and possibly some regression. Autism is a chronic condition, so it's often two steps forward, and one back. Are you better this year compared to last year? Day to day is too variable; think month-to-month and year-to-year. Compare your son to how he was this same time last year, as weather, allergens, and temperatures can cause interim disruptions; year to year is the best indicator of a favorable trend. And don't count on yourself to notice and remember progress—or lack thereof—keep careful notes. You'll often find yourself thinking, "Wow—I had forgotten that he used to do that."

KEY TIP

Keep some sort of journal of therapies and treatments along with reactions. I have a spreadsheet for this that you can download at www.skyhorsepublishing.com/book/?GCOI-60239108168770&. Update this (or a similar log) daily, and over time, you will be able to see what is working, and share this information with your doctor and therapists.

~

Younger kids may respond quicker, but do not give up if they don't. Also, kids are never too old to start. Plus, you never know what treatments will become available; there are new therapies to try every year. Keep breathing and moving forward!

~

Be open-minded when choosing among the various therapies; remember the proverb of the "empty cup":

> A learned man once went to visit a Zen teacher to inquire about Zen. As the Zen teacher talked, the learned man frequently interrupted to express his own opinion about this or that.
>
> Finally, the Zen teacher stopped talking and began to serve tea to the learned man. He poured the cup full, then kept pouring until the cup overflowed.

"Stop," said the learned man. "The cup is full; no more can be poured in."

"Like this cup, you are full of your own opinions," replied the Zen teacher. "If you do not first empty your cup, how can you taste my tea?"

Supplements

When giving supplements, it's best to teach your son to take pills/capsules, but in the interim, utilize liquids, powders, and chewables as available (most come in multiple formulations). Anything in a capsule can be mixed into food or drink.

To encourage your son to take pills/capsules: Use rewards to entice him to take his caps. Our kids usually have something they go absolutely bonkers over, so use it for good. You should also be firm about taking the caps; let him know that it will happen. It's not open to negotiation. To do this, don't try and fool him by hiding the cap in, say, applesauce. I give Alex his supplements on top of the applesauce, so he knows what he's getting; the applesauce is just there to help make it easier.

~

So what if your kid doesn't swallow pills? There are two important keys to success with this, the roux and the meat injector! Empty all your capsules into a small cup with highish sides (I use a 3 oz. Tupperware container), add any additional powders. Then add a tiny bit of liquid (I use filtered water or liquid molybdenum, depending on whether it is morning or evening)—just enough to make a roux (or thick paste), if you add too much liquid, the powders will clump and you will have a mess. Stir it thoroughly so it has an even consistency then add more water to almost fill the cup. Next comes the meat injector! Use a meat injector instead of a syringe (a syringe is at most 2T, a meat injector holds much more liquid)—you can purchase one at Bed Bath and Beyond or any store that carries cooking tools. Remove the needle, suck up the supplement stew and squirt it into your child's mouth.

—Peggy Becker, National Autism Association
—New York Metro, Vice President

If using powders or breaking open caps, you can mix into foods or try making a smoothie. It's a good way to get some nice antioxidant berries and other good stuff down with the supplements at the same time.

~

Some prescribed meds may only be available compounded, or they are easier to use in a compound form. Just remember that if you have Medicaid for your son, the compounding pharmacy has to be in your home state, or else Medicaid will not cover it (it's a state program).

Home Remedies

Activated charcoal (AC) lessens the die-offs associated with antifungal treatments and other detox therapies by absorbing chemicals/waste. AC also serves to help with any GI disturbances (even hangovers), use it yourself and see. Just remember to give two hours before or after other meds/supplements, as it will not discriminate in what it absorbs and removes. More on AC from WebMD:

> Common charcoal is made from peat, coal, wood, coconut shell, or petroleum. "Activated charcoal" is similar to common charcoal, but is made especially for use as a medicine. To make activated charcoal, manufacturers heat common charcoal in the presence of a gas that causes the charcoal to develop lots of internal spaces or "pores." These pores help activated charcoal "trap" chemicals.
>
> Activated charcoal is used to treat poisonings, reduce intestinal gas (flatulence), lower cholesterol levels, prevent hangover, and treat bile flow problems (cholestasis) during pregnancy.

~

Epsom salt baths act as a natural detoxifier and also aid in constipation and help calming. The one occasional negative can be dry skin; if your child experiences dry skin, just add some baking soda to the mix. This is one of the easiest therapies to try.

Constipation

When dealing with constipation, remember one good "cleaning" is not all it takes. In most cases it took your child years to develop the condition, you need to get him regular for months to shrink the colon back to size.

~

For handling constipation there are a number of reliable and safe non-medical alternatives including supplementing magnesium (consult a physician for dosage), aloe juice (pour a little into the morning juice) and Fruit-Eze, which is a prune, raisin, and date jam. If your child doesn't like the taste, you can cover it with something like peanut butter or syrup.

Gastrointestinal (GI) Troubles

So many, if not most kids on the spectrum have GI issues, from dietary allergens to full-blown Irritable Bowel Disease (IBD). My son Alex has ulcerative colitis, which went undetected for years, treatment of which has benefited not only his GI tract but his autism as well.

~

If your child has frequent nighttime awakenings and/ or wettings, they should have a full GI workup; nighttime awakenings can mean reflux, and wettings can mean allergies.

~

The presence of chronic (i.e., long-standing) GI symptoms demands medical evaluation. The fact that the child has autism is merely an interesting sidebar item. The symptoms typically consist of any (or all) of the following:

- Abdominal pain
- Diarrhea (defined as unformed stool that does not hold its own shape but rather conforms to the shape of the container/nappy/diaper that it is in)
- Constipation (defined as infrequent passage of stool of any consistency or passage of overly hard stools regardless of frequency)
- Soft-stool constipation
- Painful passage of unformed stool
- Rectal prolapse
- Failure to maintain normal growth
- Regurgitation
- Rumination
- Abdominal distention
- Food avoidance

> —Dr. Arthur Krigsman, "Gastrointestinal Disease: Emerging Consensus," Cutting-Edge Therapies for Autism

~

Parents, physicians, and therapists must realize that difficult-to-treat ASD behaviors or behaviors that have not been responsive to standard behavioral interventions might be the sole manifestation of a GI diagnosis. This means that unprovoked aggression, violent behavior, and irritability might have an underlying GI cause, and this must be taken into consideration prior to the reflexive desire to begin a psychotropic drug such as risperidone (despite its FDA approval for the treatment of autism).

—*Dr. Arthur Krigsman, "Gastrointestinal Disease: Emerging Consensus,"* Cutting-Edge Therapies for Autism

~

Gastroesophageal reflux disease, gastritis/gastric ulcer, and constipation are just three examples of GI diagnoses that are known to cause behavioral symptoms. In addition, poor focus and an inability to make significant academic or communicative progress despite intensive interventions might indicate the presence of treatable bowel disease that, once treated, can significantly improve the child's degree of disability.

—*Dr. Arthur Krigsman, "Gastrointestinal Disease: Emerging Consensus,"* Cutting-Edge Therapies for Autism

Medications

Before filling a drug prescription, ask a lot of questions, especially ones like: Are there any possible side effects? Will his sleep be affected? What is in the actual formulation? How exactly does it work on my child's mind? Also ask about the success/non-success rate, as this is usually important when it comes to letting you know how effective the drug may be for your child's particular needs. Medications are not something to be treated lightly without regard.

Symptoms such as aggression and self-injurious behavior are often responses to pain. Before assuming a psychological genesis, be 100 percent certain that your child is not in pain. In particular, stomach pain and/or gastroesophageal reflux should be ruled out.

The Autism Research Institute has surveyed more than 27,000 parents since 1967; often-prescribed meds like Risperdal, Ritalin, and Prozac are by no means the most successful treatments. Before choosing psychotropic meds that often have unpleasant side effects, consider dietary intervention. Read ARI's survey: (autism.com/pdf/providers/ParentRatings2009.pdf), and consider biomedical treatment. Make sure all educational therapies are appropriately implemented.

~

Signs that would alert you to the need for medication management include:

- Your child's safety is being questioned
- Increased episodes of physical aggression toward self and others

- Episodes of physical or verbal aggression are prolonged and not responsive to other intervention techniques
- Uncontrolled temper tantrums
- Fear that your child will hurt you or other members of your family or support team
- Increase in repetitive or stereotypic behaviors despite other interventions being in place
- Increase in anxiety, impulsivity, and inattention despite other interventions being in place

> —*Dr. Mark Freilich, "Pharmaceutical Medication Management: The Why, When, and What,"* Cutting-Edge Therapies for Autism

The process of determining the appropriate medication and the appropriate dosage cannot be completed overnight. The process will, at first, require weekly office visits (or at least weekly telephone communication) with the prescribing physician. If, at any point before finding the "optimal" dosage, the physician hands you a prescription and tells you that the plan is to administer the medication and return in a month's time, please consider another medication manager.

> —*Dr. Mark Freilich, "Pharmaceutical Medication Management: The Why, When, and What,"* Cutting-Edge Therapies for Autism

~

Antibiotics should be used sparingly and only for confirmed bacterial infections (they do not alleviate viral infections). Remember, antibiotic use disrupts the normal gut flora and promotes the overgrowth of yeast and resistant organisms that, in turn, harms the optimal functioning of the immune system. Bear in mind that most ear infections are viral and are thus not treatable with antibiotics. Use homeopathic eardrops to help ease the symptoms associated with ear infections and colds. And if antibiotics are required, utilize a good probiotic to help offset the loss of gut flora.

Vaccinations

A touchy subject for some, I will simply state better safe than sorry. Here are some suggestions that are just common sense.

- If your child has a fever, constipation, diarrhea, or other illness, hold off on the vaccination.
- If your child is on antibiotics, hold off on the vaccination.
- If your child has an immune system disorder, allergies, or if they had a reaction to an earlier vaccine, hold off on the vaccine and seek another opinion.
- Know what the possible reactions are to each vaccine given.
- Immediately report side effects to your doctor.
- Remember to ask for single-dose preservative free (mercury-free) vaccines.

- Break up the measles, mumps, rubella (MMR) shot and give those months apart.
- Check antibody titers before boosters, as they (the boosters) may not be necessary. Vaccination is a medical procedure after all and no need to take on unnecessary risk.

Here is the recommended vaccine schedule of Stephanie Cave, MD, vaccine expert:

- Birth: Hepatitis B (only if mom is Hepatitis B positive); otherwise, no vaccine shot
- 4 months: Hib, IPV
- 5 months: DTaP
- 6 months: Hib, IPV
- 7 months: DTaP
- 8 months: Hib
- 9 months: DTaP
- 15 months: Measles
- 17 months: Hib, IPV
- 18 months: DTaP
- 24 months: Prevnar (1 dose only)
- 27 months: Rubella
- 30 months: Mumps
- 4 years: Varicella (if not immune already)
- 4 to 5 years: Hepatitis B series
- 4 to 5 years: DTaP, IPV boosters

- 4 to 5 years: Test titers for MMR and do not give unless not immune. Immunize only for vaccines found to be negative.

NOTE: If your pediatrician has a problem with these requests, choose another doctor. Consider, when infants are developing pediatricians remind parents to wait months to years to introduce certain foods (solids, dairy, eggs, fish, nuts, etc.) to watch for and help avoid allergic reactions, yet also recommend than many of the vaccinations on the schedule be given at once. Ask them why this makes sense if there is resistance to the above.

First Aid

Having a first aid kit at home is of absolute necessity along with knowing how to use it. Take a class in first aid at your local firehouse or medical facility and you may be able to save a visit to the doctor or other such facility that can be traumatic for our kids.

~

To adjust to minor cuts and scrapes let your child play wear a band-aid now and then so the actual need is no big deal. Let them practice on you. Wear a band-aid yourself, or if there is a chronic issue try to mimic what they will have to deal with so that they can become a bit more comfortable with the process.

Preparing for that Inevitable Doctor/Emergency Room Visit

When visiting the doctor or other related facility bring along something comforting for the child, such as a favorite toy or blanket or perhaps a device (iPad). Anything to keep him busy and not have to focus exclusively on the stress of visiting a medical establishment. It may be useful to visit said establishment in advance to familiarize the child and remove one level of stress—the unknown.

Likewise, watch some shows that have a nice comfortable perspective going to see medical personnel. Again this helps your child become familiar with the process and see that things will be ok.

~

Play doctor with your child to familiarize him with what goes on in the medical office to ease stress. Give each other a play examination, perhaps when you visit the doctor they can let your child listen to the stethoscope or hold a dental mirror and raise and lower the examination table/chair to gain their trust.

~

Walk around the facility with your kid. There will be restrictions to this of course but in my experience staff at medical facilities are usually well-versed on autism and the anxiety kids can experience. A little tour can help.

Older Kids

Although many tips in this book state that early intervention brings better outcomes, this should not, and is not meant to, discourage those of you whose children are older (which includes myself). Biomedical and every other therapeutic approach can be started at any age, including teens and adults. I have heard many stories of people with autism at all ages showing significant improvement with various therapies. Most of Alex's progress to date has come after the age of fourteen.

Finding Help

Find a biomedical "maven," someone already ahead of you on the learning curve. This could be another parent you know, someone from a parent social group, or your son's school. If you cannot find someone nearby that you trust, you can contact organizations such as the National Autism Association (NAA), Talk About Curing Autism (TACA), or Generation Rescue (GR). All have lists of parents who are biomedical mavens and donate their time to talk to parents who are new to the approach. Check out the NAA and GR sites. NAA calls their mavens Naavigators and GR calls them Rescue Angels.

Chapter 4

Financial

"Buy what you do not need, and soon you will sell your necessities."

—Benjamin Franklin

Making Ends Meet

Virtually all families with an autistic child struggle financially, I am no exception. I'd like to tell you there is a secret fund for ASDs or some magical account that covers therapies, but there just is not. You will be challenged and forced to make tough financial calls. What I can and do provide are solid financial planning Tips from my own experience and from other experts to help cushion the blows. *Note to parents, the ABLE (Achieving a Better Life Experience) tax-free accounts were just passed and signed into law; we will not review here as details are to come, but ask your financial planner/accountant about this new option.*

~

While there is some help from the government, most notably Medicaid, there is not nearly enough. Your child

43

may qualify for Supplemental Security Income (SSI), but this and Medicaid benefits will only go so far. You will likely dip, if not drain, savings and borrow from any deep pockets, especially if you pursue biomedical and alternative therapies, most of which are not covered by any insurance. For the best outcomes you will need an intensive (read: expensive) program and will have to make decisions that will not necessarily be sound from a financial perspective. Just remember that things will only get more expensive in the long run without progress so though it may seem challenging financially to create an intensive program, in the long run you will benefit.

~

KEY TIP

Once your son is diagnosed as autistic, or anyplace on the spectrum, he is entitled to Medicaid. Google "Medicaid Waiver Programs" in your home state, and you will find organizations that will walk you through the application process, free of charge, and educate you as to just what benefits are included with the waiver programs.

~

You may also find additional resources through state or local laws that are designed to help children with handicaps (which includes autism, but may not specify as such—for instance, handicapped parking). Research available services provided for your child in your immediate area to obtain maximum benefits, talk to parent "mavens," and ask your local state representatives; they are eager to help their constituents.

Tax Tips by Kim Mack Rosenberg and Mark L. Berger, CPA

The information contained herein is for informational purposes only and does not substitute for tax advice from your own tax adviser, familiar with your financial information. While they have endeavored to be as accurate as possible, the authors make no warranties, express or implied, concerning the information contained herein. As always, official sources and publications and your own tax professional should be consulted for the most current rules and regulations that may be applicable to you.

- Medical expenses above the first 7.5 percent of your adjusted gross income are tax-deductible. Medical expenses up to the first 7.5 percent of adjusted gross income are never deductible (even when your expenses exceed 7.5 percent of your adjusted gross income; only the excess is deductible).
- Save medical receipts for your entire family, even if you don't think you will qualify for a medical

---

expense deduction. You never know when a catastrophic medical bill or a change in family finances could happen and put you over the 7.5 percent threshold.

- IRS publication 502, available at www.IRS.gov, is a great resource to determine what is deductible. Pub. 502 also lists expenses that generally are not deductible, but exceptions in those categories often allow deductions for some of the medical care required by special-needs children.

- Get a letter from a doctor(s) substantiating your child's need for his treatments and related expenses, like occupational therapy, physical therapy, speech therapy, supplements, special toys/equipment, homeopathy, hyperbaric treatment, the need for you to attend conferences/buy books related to your child's condition or treatment, typical classes (for socialization, for example, if essential to your child's treatment). If you make this an easy step for your practitioners, they are usually amenable to helping you—they want your child to get the treatments he or she needs, too! Keep this letter in case of audit.

- Supplements that are recommended by a medical practitioner to treat a medical condition diagnosed by a doctor may be deductible, but supplements taken for general "good health" reasons are not deductible.

- Tuition for a therapeutic school generally will qualify as a medical expense, but if you are reimbursed for that tuition in a later tax year, you will have to account for the reimbursement, and, under some circumstances, some portion could count as income. Reimbursements (including insurance reimbursements) are taxable to the extent that the expense was deducted. If you don't deduct the tuition and then don't get reimbursed, you have three years from the date that you filed that year's return to go back and amend your return.

- For car travel for medical purposes, you can deduct the larger of the statutory mileage rate (it changes each year and is different for medical vs. business) or your actual expenses (gas and oil, primarily). Tolls and parking are deductible in addition to either actual costs or the statutory per mile deduction. If you use your car in connection with medical expenses and take the standard medical mileage rate deduction, you should keep a mileage log (you can even keep it in the car to be sure to have it when you need it).

- Conference fees and transportation expenses for conferences you attend to learn about your child's medical condition/treatment are includable medical expenses; however, meals and lodging at the conference are not.

- The cost of travel (including an accompanying parent's costs) to another city for medical care is deductible if the primary purpose of your trip is to treat a medical condition. Lodging (at a statutorily defined rate) also is deductible when traveling out of town for medical treatment.

- However, meals are not deductible (except for the patient in a hospital or similar facility).

- The difference between the cost of foods for special diets (such as the gluten-free/casein-free diet) versus "normal" equivalents is deductible when the special diet is prescribed by a doctor to alleviate a medical condition. For a handy template on these sometimes-complicated calculations, check out www.TACAnow.org.

- You should evaluate employer-provided plans such as a flex-spending plan, because it gives you the opportunity to pay for medical expenses with pre-tax earnings.

- Medical expenses reimbursed by a flex spending plan do not qualify as medical expenses for tax deduction purposes—you paid for this with pre-tax dollars and cannot "double dip." (In other words, if you were reimbursed by flex spending, you cannot claim the expense on your taxes).

- Insurance premiums paid with pre-tax dollars (which is the case for many employees) are not deductible. If you are self-employed, these premiums may be subject to different tax treatment (not as a medical expense).

- In balancing flex-spending dollars vs. insurance coverage, if you think an expense may be covered by your insurance, submit it to your insurer first. Use your flex spending dollars wisely.

- Expenses not covered by insurance and not tax deductible may still be eligible for flex spending. These items even include some OTC medications. Consult your flex spending account information on reimbursable items. If you can use pre-tax dollars to be repaid for items that are not tax-deductible, it might make sense to use flex-spending dollars for those items before potentially tax-deductible items.

- Payments for medical expenses necessary to meet your insurance policy deductible as well as co-pays after you meet your deductible are tax-deductible.

- The best practice is to keep receipts and to document everything in case of an audit.

- Documentation of medical expenses should include the name and address of the person you paid and the amount and date you paid, a description of the service/goods provided, and the date provided.

- Try not to pay medical expenses with cash—credit cards and checks are easier to substantiate.

- If your child/family has a lot of medical expenses, stay on top of filing regularly. If your paperwork builds up, items may go missing and the task becomes too daunting. Create a filing system that works for you.

- Submit each claim to your insurer separately, one claim per envelope. Claims are less likely to be lost if they arrive separately rather than in bulk.

- Keep a copy of the claim form and provider's bill/receipt in case the insurer misplaces the claim and you need to resubmit, and to help you keep track of paid and outstanding claims. Note the date you sent it on your copy. When you receive an explanation of benefits from your insurer, you can attach it to these documents.

- Learn how to read your insurer's "explanation of benefits" to determine what is tax-deductible on a given claim and to be sure you are accounting for all potential deductions. Any deduction is based on what remains after the charge is reduced based on any agreement your doctor or other provider may have with the insurer, and after your insurer pays its share. These may include: "not covered amounts"; co-pays; deductibles; and co-insurance (for example, if you have a 70/30 plan—your 30 percent share of the allowed charge is a deductible medical expense).

- To help you and your tax preparer prepare your return efficiently and accurately, create a document (in a word processing, database, or spreadsheet program with which you are comfortable), or use a money management program that allows you to track the expenses by category or groups of categories. If you create a document, you can use the same document and save it as a new version each year—no need to reinvent the wheel.

Tax Related

While reviewing your taxes, should you notice a benefit that you missed claiming in past years, you may file an amended return within three years of the date that you filed the original return.

~

Additional caregivers, such as grandparents, aunts and uncles, and even non-relative caregivers, may qualify for tax benefits through various means. Be sure to mention any funds used to help the child (even if not your own) to your tax preparer. Please make sure you meet the requirements, though, as this is pretty tightly regulated by the IRS.

~

Ask your son's various physicians, therapists, and other professionals for a letter stating what treatments, therapies, and or meds they require on an annual basis and file it. Should the IRS audit you regarding medical expense deductions, these letters will prove invaluable.

Insurance

When paying for medical expenses, utilize the bucket system:

- **Bucket One:** Insurance/Medicaid; if the expense is not covered, then use

- **Bucket Two:** Flexible Spending Accounts; if not eligible (or if they are already used up), then use
- **Bucket Three:** Medical Expense Deduction. If it can be deemed a "good medical expense," save it for tax season.

~

Remember that insurance is a business—your provider wants to take in more money than it pays out. This is definitely an area in which the squeaky wheel gets the grease.

~

While you will likely need to rearrange your work schedule or even your career, keep in mind that one parent should keep a good insurance plan, either from an employer or through some association. Medical costs and therapies are very expensive, and while there have been some improvements in various laws (notably in the coverage of ABA) many therapies remain uncovered. Remember that once your child has an official diagnosis they are entitled to Medicaid, which has pros and cons but can frequently provide some help. Many points on this are covered throughout the book.

Special Needs Trust

A special needs trust (SNT) serves two primary functions: First, it provides management of funds for your son should he not be able to do so himself, and second, it preserves your son's eligibility for public benefits, including Medicaid, SSI, or any other program. Below are some SNT Tips.

- The SNT allows you to leave resources for his benefit without cutting off public assistance (Medicaid and such) and ensures that your other children will not be overburdened with his care.

- You may think you do not need a SNT currently, but remember that things change; public programs change over the years, and siblings may have their own difficulties. A SNT can provide a secure future for your son.

- To create the SNT you will need the help of a lawyer with experience in SNTs. Ask other parents for references; contact your Medicaid coordinator, as these organizations sometimes provide discounted or free legal help. Ask your current lawyers covering other areas of your life for a referral.

- Together with your legal and financial advisors, you will choose an appropriate trustee who will manage the SNT.

- When meeting with the above professionals, assess your current situation, analyze the impact of the plan on your estate and aid programs, and then adjust as necessary.

Financial

Teaching Your Son Money 101
by Joseph Campagna

There is an old saying in teaching, "meet the child where they are." I don't profess to be a teacher but I was a child (maybe I still am to a certain extent).

I did well in school but never excelled to my potential (so I was told). However, I enjoy reading and learning what interests me or I need to know. Maybe that makes me average.

I think when relating personal accounts, it is extremely important for our population to have a proper background so the reader can put his/her situation in perspective. I have read many positive stories (and I applaud everyone's success) only to realize that the account wasn't relative to my son because of the different level of the affected child. I secretly would kill for an Asperger's diagnosis for my son!

My son, Chris, is sixteen years old. He has a PDD-NOS diagnosis and he is verbal. He is somewhere at a 3rd–4th grade academic level. He struggles with social interaction and is prone to scripting and some stimming. He has come a long way from the days of nearly constant disregulation and running into Madison Avenue. We live with my wife, daughter, and our dog on the upper east side of Manhattan.

So now let's start . . .

The only two motivators for my son are food and videos. Yet, I see a bit (if not more) of myself in him. One similarity is that we are practical learners. In growing up with humble means in Long Island, NY, I was raised with an allowance. In today's parlance it may be called "pay for performance." It motivated me because my Dad's view was "you can do/ have anything you want, if you can pay for it." Even forty years ago, the initial $5 a week didn't go far. Yet, it was pocket money and since it was not much it instilled a desire for taking on odd jobs in my later teen years. So we have introduced a $20 a week allowance with Chris. For his daily "jobs" he has some basic hygiene tasks, he has to make his bed, take out the garbage, unload the dishwasher, and feed the dog. I would say he completes tasks about 80 percent of the time without prompting and 99 percent with prompting.

CHRIS "GETS" MONEY! It empowers him to buy goods and services he wants. Typically we will go to the diner on Saturday mornings either across 96th St (a busy street) from our apartment or in the next town over from Grandma's house in rural Connecticut. Chris must use his money (which can be a mix of his allowance or gifts, i.e., birthday) to buy his breakfast. Once breakfast is done, we do "menu math." He must tally his bill from the menu (I allow him to use his iPhone calculator but have also done it without the calculator) and then make change. Some days are better than others but on the whole he is pretty good. We have been trying to have Chris carry ID for years in a wallet but he had no interest. However, with his money now he will keep the wallet with his iPhone in his backpack, which he takes almost everywhere. An added benefit is that when we go shopping (i.e., groceries and/ or Target) he knows that I will not buy him anything extra so he has to use his wallet money. This puts a natural cap on what I call 'the shopping begging." It also works for my neuro-typical daughter!

We expanded our diner routine by having Chris walk to the diner himself, which required him to solo across 96th St. Logistically, we live across the street one way from the diner (96th St.) and the other way from Starbucks (Madison Avenue). Our Citibank branch is three doors down from the diner. Chris can be somewhat rigid in his behavior but one upside is he NEVER crosses a street at the red signal. This gave me confidence to try and let him go to the bank and the diner by himself and then meet him. While I pondered the proposition for months, I finally mustered the courage.

First, I asked Chris if he wanted to go by himself, to which he overwhelmingly agreed. Then I explained we would leave together and I would go to Starbucks and meet him at the diner. The Starbucks location has large windows by which I watched Chris navigate the street corner. I will be honest, it was the longest time I have ever held my breath! He did fine. Once he was across, I went outside to the street corner where I could see him at the Citibank door. He had some trouble with the card reader but eventually got in when someone exited. Staying relatively discreet, I watched him come out and go to the diner. When I arrived at the diner, he was seated in our normal booth like it was any other day. We have a great relationship with the diner staff as we have been going there for over ten years. They know about Chris's dairy allergy and they have my cell phone number should Chris go to the diner on his own. Frankly, I haven't used that option more because I like to go with him.

I am looking to build upon the diner experience into a supported employment opportunity. Last week I asked the manager if Chris could do a couple hours a week as a busboy. He said he would ask the owner. I also went to the local high school to get Chris his working papers. It was a relatively easy process to complete the form and bring some documentation. We'll see . . .

We have expanded the money concept to banking. Prior to sixteen years old, he couldn't have his own account. So I opened another account under my name with a separate ATM card. It's linked to our main account so we can avoid monthly fees by keeping a combined minimum balance. We do not keep over $100 in the account and we can transfer money via computer or ATM. After some training, Chris can now manage the card reader to enter Citibank and use his PIN to withdraw money. He takes the same amount each time so it's pretty rote but he is proficient. Also, I fully expected to be getting at least a handful of replacement ATM cards by now and in the year and a half that we have had the account, no replacement cards have been required.

Financial

We have some stretch goals going forward:

- supported employment
- navigating the bus for local trips
- accessing the bank account via his iPhone
- using his iPhone more

Here are a few things to keep in mind:

- Inventory your child's strengths and try to build opportunities based on them (Chris never crosses at a red street signal)
- Augment familiar people and places to expand autonomous behaviors (Chris loves the diner)
- Key into your child's motivators and use tools to empower them and create teachable moments (the power of money and menu math)
- Trust your own experience (an allowance worked in my childhood)
- You can't trust someone, until you trust them. This always involves the risk of an unknown outcome. This is especially so for our population but also even more important. Try to structure a new experience in a way that can get you comfortable with the risk (supervising crossing the street from Starbucks)

As with any advice, if makes sense, try it. If it works, great! If not, try something else. Certainly, one size does NOT fit all.

Chapter 5

Educational

Education is not the learning of facts, but the training of the mind to think.

—Albert Einstein

Back to School

As a parent, remember you are in charge. You have the power. View yourself as CEO of your child's programs, with education being one division. If you are not getting the results you desire, make a change. Parents have more influence than they tend to believe with school systems.

Early Intervention

For early intervention services, if a child is under the age of three, call your local early intervention agency. Check your state's Developmental Disability Agency for more information at www.ddrcco.com/states.htm.

~

Children ages zero to three and school-age children might be eligible for speech and language services through the state in which they reside. Government agencies within your state will be able to provide contact information to begin the assessment process, which will determine eligibility for services. School-age children might be evaluated to determine the need for speech-language therapy within the school setting. In addition, licensed therapists in your area can be located by visiting the American Speech-Language-Hearing Association (ASHA) website (www.ASHA.org), asking your child's doctor, or by contacting local support groups and agencies.

—*Lavinia Pereira and Michelle Solomon, "Speech-Language Therapy,"* Cutting-Edge Therapies for Autism

Dealing with School

Collect emails from your son's teacher, principal, VPs, superintendent, chancellor, etc. When you email concerns, cc as many senior folks as possible on the email. This can help motivate some in what is typically a bureaucratic system, and creates a proper paper trail. Likewise, if you have good things to say, do the same. Show that you are informed, will take action, and comment. The squeaky wheel gets greased may not be your style, but it's effective in this type of environment and it regards your child, so cc away.

~

When speaking to your son's Board of Education (BOE), remember the phrase, "appropriate education." Your son is entitled by the Individuals with Disabilities Education Act (IDEA) to a free appropriate public education. If your BOE cannot provide one, they must cover the cost of an APPROPRIATE private school. Appropriate does not mean best. Keep this in mind. The Supreme Court interprets an appropriate education plan as one that "must be reasonably calculated to provide educational benefit to the individual child."

Do not hesitate to question the "plan." IEPs are once per year, but ideally your child will improve on a more frequent basis, so call for a meeting if the current IEP is no longer relevant or appropriate.

~

Should you believe a private school is the best option, and you'll miss the $60,000 to $100,000 they cost, you will need an education lawyer. *Education Lawyer.* Not uncle Steve or your next-door neighbor who happens to be an attorney. For this you need a specialist. Ask your target school, as they likely have a list of lawyers other parents use. Interview a few and choose the one you like, and ask for parent references.

~

Keep a positive pattern of communication with teachers/ school. I email the school each morning on how Alex is doing and did the night before, noting any issues to watch out for and asking for feedback.

So keep a solid professional, consistent relationship with teachers/school. Note the good things, maybe give a small holiday gift, but do not hesitate to say or note problems or issues of concern. I have come across resistance. But, with a bit of a push, I have done what's been needed and done it with respect.

~

In those daily emails/notes, inform school about any troubles at home that may impact the day. Say the child did not sleep his normal eight last night, or had a meltdown getting ready for school.

Inform staff about your child. Though they may have diagnoses and paperwork, let's face it, all kids on the spectrum are different and you are the expert. Tell them your child's unique wants, needs, skills, and strengths.

~

NOTE: It is illegal for a public school to tell parents that their child cannot come back to school unless on medication. Not so in private school.

Finding the Right Fit

When looking at schools, focus on the right educational and therapeutic environment for your son. The right educational program in an overcrowded, busy school will not help your son in the long run if he has significant sensory issues. A smaller, soothing class might accomplish more than the educational program itself. Overall, choose the environment that will allow your son to function at his best.

~

Questions to ask when you visit a recommended program:

- What is the educational philosophy of the program (ABA, DIR, TEAACH)?
- What is the class size and ratio to teachers/teaching assistants?
- How long has the school been using the current program (ABA, DIR, etc.)?
- How do the nonverbal kids communicate?
- What kind of success has the program had (i.e., kids moving to less-restrictive classes)?
- What programs are offered to parents?
- How long have the teachers taught at this school?
- What is their experience with kids with autism?
- How are related services provided?
- What services are currently being provided to students in the class?
- Does the school have a consultant or supervisor certified in the particular philosophy?

- Does the consultant/supervisor conduct ongoing training for school staff?
- What is the age makeup of the class? (NOTE: There can only be a three-year age span in each class.)
- Where do the special education kids have lunch and recreation?
- Are there inclusion opportunities?
- How does the staff handle behavioral issues and/or self-injurious behaviors?
- What types of reinforcers are used at the school?
- Is medical staff available at the school?
- Don't forget to observe a class and take copious notes!

~

Consider moving to another state. Some states spend a greater percentage of their budgets on social services and thus have more services available. These states tend to have a higher percentage of children with autism as well, so there are more parents to network with and likely more specialized schools. Put politics aside, because you need all the help you can get; seek out those states friendliest to the "autism family." Easter Seals has compiled a list titled State Autism Profiles: www.easterseals.com/explore-resources/living-with-autism/state-autism-profiles.html. Check it out and see where your state ranks.

~

Consider choosing a school in which your child will not be noticeably more "peculiar" than everyone else; children can be harsh critics. Children who attend learning-disabled schools are often more accepting of differences in others; even if they are simply dyslexic, they often place less value on conformity.

~

In school, your son's class should have almost as many teachers and assistants as kids. If he is at the high-functioning end of the spectrum, focus on mainstreaming and having typical peer interactions. If on the more challenged end of the spectrum, focus on a high teacher-student ratio and large amounts of therapy time.

~

It is often an educational goal for parents and professionals for a child to be mainstreamed. While an important goal, it is more important to consider your child's feelings of competence in these settings. Typical role models can be good, but the reality is that children's interactions are full of innuendo. Academically, your child may be able to keep up with a mainstream class, but socially, he or she is likely lagging behind. Ask yourself: are these role models providing positive experiences for my child, or is my child feeling bullied, isolated, or incompetent in that environment?

—Laura Hynes, LMSW, RDI Program Certified Consultant

The Communication Behavior Link

Remember that behavior is communication. If a nonverbal child has no communication system, they will learn to communicate inappropriate behaviors. Often educators and parents are hesitant to use alternative systems of communications (i.e., PECS, typing, sign language) because they are afraid it will hinder speech developing, or that it is like giving up on their child or student. However, research has proven just the opposite: these alternative communication methods enhance the child's ability to speak.

—*Chantal Sicile-Kira, author of* Autism Life Skills

~

"If a functional communication system has not been put into place with a child, his only recourse is behavior."

—*Temple Grandin.*

Facilitating Communication

Make your own PECS. I took photos of my son's favorite foods, activities, and places. Using iPhoto or a similar program, you can arrange and order wallet-sized photos to place into a photo book or business card holder for easy access at home and on the road.

~

If you just hand over a snack item, there is no opportunity to discuss . . . anything! But put two different kinds of snacks in a clear bag, and you create an opportunity for discussion before your child eats.

~

KEY TIP

I can actually call this Tip a game changer for those of us with non-verbal kids. Simply, get an iPad. There are several great communication apps now available now, including Proloquo2go™, AutisMate and Avatalker (www. avatalkeraac.com). Also, if you child is non-verbal you can have your local BOE cover the cost of the device, including devices that become damaged, along with the price of protective covers (for this I recommend OtterBox, the Defender series). Below is a short speech I gave about how the iPad has helped Alex and some other helpful information in regards to the device.

February 27, 2014—Apple Store, SoHo NYC

My son, Alex is a non-verbal fifteen-year-old boy with autism. Alex presently attends public school here in Manhattan. He has used an iPad for well over 3 years now and favors the use of YouTube for entertainment and Proloquo2Go™, which is his primary means of communication. Tonight, I am going to share how this technology has helped Alex in the areas of frustration and independence. I'll also discuss how you can have the government, in the form of the BOE (Board of Education) or Medicaid (waiver reimbursement) cover the cost of what they call—a Dynamic Display Speech Generating Device. Yes, that is what the iPad is referred to on an IEP. Only a government bureaucrat could turn "iPad" into "Dynamic Display Speech Generating Device."

Frustration: Before the iPad came along, Alex had to rely on gestures, approximations, and PECS images to communicate his needs and wants. As you can imagine, this is quite an inefficient means of communication and led to tremendous frustration for Alex and his caregivers. Especially when he was feeling ill, hungry, or if someone other than myself was with him. In these trying circumstances Alex would frequently melt down and even turn aggressive towards himself and or his caregiver as he became exasperated with his inability to convey his requirements.

Since getting his iPad, this has dissipated tremendously (I estimate at least 90 percent) as he can now communicate with ease to anyone his wants, needs, and feelings. Also, I and Alex's caregivers now realize just how much Alex truly understands, how great his receptive skills are, and how truly smart he is, and this is reflected in his greater level of confidence at home and in school.

Independence: Having an iPad has led to a measure of independence for Alex, as prior to, Alex needed others to help him be entertained when indoors, whether it was putting the TV on, loading videos, setting up computer games, etc. Now Alex can do all this himself on his iPad and he is motivated to do so thanks to the ease and logic of the device.

Alex over these three years has now become more communicative in general thanks to the success he now has in getting his points across. This has also led to his "sounds," meaning his word approximations, to become gradually clearer, which is very exciting to me. In fact, earlier today, Alex was working with his speech therapist and he clearly enunciated "milk," for almond milk, for the first time!

Coverage: Alex has his iPad and app paid for and covered via the BOE. He brings the device to school, home, wherever he needs it, so he has a consistent voice and access to his favorite programs. The way this works, is, you have your child evaluated to "confirm" they are non-verbal or would benefit from a device. Once this is confirmed, for example on a student's IEP, then the BOE or Medicaid is required to cover the cost of the device and app.

To get a specific app or device (as there are options), you can have the child evaluated on the desired device/app. So in Alex's case, I asked the BOE technology team to test him on an iPad, he easily manipulated and maneuvered through the test, and now he has a free device. Which I should mention is replaced by the BOE whenever damaged, as has happened a couple of times in our case (a protective case is also available under this coverage as requested).

So if you are working with a child or have a child who can benefit from this technology, check with your school/therapist/social worker on getting the device and apps covered.

To conclude, the iPad has been a real game changer for us. It has given Alex a voice, and let myself and others know just how much he truly understands, and provided him a measure of independence and confidence.

Communication Tips from Temple

The tips in this section come from Temple Grandin, PhD, author of *Thinking in Pictures* and *The Way I See It*; www.autism.com/ind_teaching_tips.asp

Some autistic individuals do not know that speech is used for communication. Language learning can be facilitated if language exercises promote communication. If the child asks for a cup, then give him a cup. If the child asks for a plate, when he wants a cup, give him a plate. The individual needs to learn that when he says words, concrete things happen. It is easier for an individual with autism to learn that their words are wrong if the incorrect word resulted in the incorrect object.

~

Children who have difficulty understanding speech have a hard time differentiating between hard consonant sounds such as "D" in dog and "L" in log. My speech teacher helped me to learn to hear these sounds by stretching out and enunciating hard consonant sounds. Even though the child might have passed a pure-tone hearing test, he might still have difficulty hearing hard consonants. Children who talk in vowel sounds are not hearing consonants.

~

Many people with autism are visual thinkers. I think in pictures. I do not think in language. All my thoughts are like videotapes running in my imagination. Pictures are my first language, and words are my second language. Nouns were the easiest words to learn because I could make a picture in my mind of the word.

~

Avoid long strings of verbal instructions. People with autism have problems with remembering the sequence. If the child can read, write the instructions down on a piece of paper. I am unable to remember sequences. If I ask for directions at a gas station, I can only remember three steps. Directions with more than three steps have to be written down. I also have difficulty remembering phone numbers because I cannot make a picture in my mind.

~

Individuals with visual processing problems often find it easier to read if black print is printed on colored paper to reduce contrast. Try light tan, light blue, gray, or light green paper. Experiment with different colors. Avoid bright yellow—it might hurt the individual's eyes. Irlen colored glasses might also make reading easier.

~

Educational

Some autistic children will learn reading more easily with phonics, and others will learn best by memorizing whole words. I learned with phonics. My mother taught me the phonics rules and then had me sound out my words. Children with lots of echolalia will often learn best if flashcards and picture books are used so that the whole words are associated with pictures. It is important to have the picture and the printed word on the same side of the card. When teaching nouns, the child must hear you speak the word and view the picture and printed word simultaneously. An example of teaching a verb would be to hold a card that says "jump," and you would jump up and down while saying "jump."

~

Several parents have informed me that using the closed captions on the television helped their child to learn to read. The child was able to read the captions and match the printed words with spoken speech. Recording a favorite program with captions on a tape would be helpful because the tape can be played over and over again and stopped.

~

The Individuals with Disabilities Education Act (IDEA)

IDEA was passed in 1990 and is designed to provide kids with learning disabilities an appropriate education in the least restrictive environment possible. Parents are to be partners in choosing the best educational fit. To do this, parents need to become familiar with the law so they know their rights and what services are available for their children.

~

It's important to know that IDEA is in effect for your child until he graduates from high school, or at least until he reaches the age of twenty-one; after this point, services are provided on a state-by-state basis. Under IDEA, every child is entitled to a Free and Appropriate Public Education (FAPE), regardless of disability. In this context, the US Supreme Court has taken appropriate to mean that the program "must be reasonably calculated to provide educational benefit to the individual child." In addition, under IDEA, all children are to be placed in the least restrictive environment possible. Remember: special education is a service, and not a place.

~

Under the Individuals with Disabilities Education Act (IDEA), services such as speech therapy, occupational therapy, vision therapy, and behavioral therapy can be provided to the child by the school district, on the condition that it has been decided that it needs to be a part of the student's individualized program at an Individual Education Program (IEP) team meeting, and written into the IEP. Parents need to inform themselves about the school district they are in, the quality of the services, their rights, and which professional in the area is the best to provide assessments of your child.

—*Chantal Sicile-Kira, author of* Autism Spectrum Disorders*, www.chantalsicile-kira.com*

More IDEA Tips

Parent rights under IDEA include the right to ask for an evaluation of your child at any time and the right to be part of the team deciding what special education services and therapies will be provided to your child.

IDEA provides for your child to have an Individualized Education Plan (IEP) designed for his specific needs; for example, how much occupational, physical, and speech therapy will be provided.

~

The specific services to be provided are decided at the annual IEP meeting, which includes yourself, your son's teachers, various school representatives, and a parent representative. You can bring your own specialists and support folks to help you in any way (moral support, reminders, etc.).

~

It's best to consult with a specialized education attorney before attending the meeting.

~

Bring a copy of the law with you to review prior to sitting down at the meeting. It's also important to bring along any other helpful documentation. Many times, they (the state team) will incorporate what you give them.

~

Should your son not progress, you have the right to question the plan and request an IEP meeting at any time to reassess the services and service levels (say the number of speech sessions) provided.

~

If there is a conflict with the educators, you have the right to have your son reevaluated. In this case, you may want to seek out a private evaluation, which can cost from a few hundred to a few thousand dollars. If you have a Medicaid waiver, you may be able to get a free outside evaluation (or at least a discounted one). Depending on where you live, it could take a while to get an appointment, so call as early as possible.

~

Should you not come to an agreement with your son's school system, you do have the right to a due process hearing where an administrative officer or judge rules. Should it come to this, you will require the services of a lawyer. Again, it's best to have an attorney (specializing in education law, do not hire just any lawyer!) in advance of this eventuality.

~

The US Department of Education has information about federal laws and state laws. Every state has a Protection and Advocacy office, which can provide you with free information in regard to your child's rights under special education. Most offices provide these laws and your rights in simple language for the layperson, in English as well as in different languages.

Here are the key parental rights under IDEA to remember:

- Parents have the right to be informed and knowledgeable about all actions taken on behalf of their child.
- Parents have the right to participate in all meetings regarding evaluation and placement.
- Parental consent is required for evaluation and placement.
- Parents have the right to challenge educational decisions through due process procedures.

The related services your son may be entitled to include:

- Speech therapy
- Occupational therapy
- Counseling
- Nursing services—medication administration
- Transportation
- Paraprofessional—health and/or transportation paras
- Physical Therapy

The Sensory Environment at School

When I was a child, loud sounds like the school bell hurt my ears like a dentist drill hitting a nerve. Children with autism need to be protected from sounds that hurt their ears. The sounds that will cause the most problems are school bells, PA systems, buzzers on the scoreboard in the gym, and the sound of chairs scraping on the floor.

—*Temple Grandin, PhD, author of* Thinking in Pictures *and*
The Way I See It; *www.autism.com/ind_teaching_tips.asp*

~

The fear of a dreaded sound can cause bad behavior. If a
child covers his ears, it is an indicator that a certain sound
hurts his ears. Sometimes sound sensitivity to a particular
sound, such as the fire alarm, can be desensitized by
recording the sound on a tape recorder. This will allow the
child to initiate the sound and gradually increase its volume.
The child must have control of playback of the sound.

—*Temple Grandin, PhD, author of* Thinking in Pictures *and*
The Way I See It; *www.autism.com/ind_teaching_tips.asp*

~

Some children might need to be warned in advance about
fire drills.

~

Some autistic people are bothered by visual distractions
and fluorescent lights. They can see the flicker of the sixty-
cycle electricity. To avoid this problem, place the child's
desk near the window or try to avoid using fluorescent
lights. If the lights cannot be avoided, use the newest
bulbs you can get. New bulbs flicker less. The flickering
of fluorescent lights can also be reduced by putting a lamp

with an old-fashioned incandescent lightbulb next to the child's desk.

> —*Temple Grandin, PhD, author of* Thinking in Pictures *and* The Way I See It; *www.autism.com/ind_teaching_tips.asp*

~

Some hyperactive autistic children who fidget all the time will often be calmer if they are given a padded weighted vest to wear. Pressure from the garment helps to calm the nervous system. I was greatly calmed by pressure. For best results, the vest should be worn for twenty minutes and then taken off for a few minutes. This prevents the nervous system from adapting to it.

> —*Temple Grandin, PhD, author of* Thinking in Pictures *and* The Way I See It; *www.autism.com/ind_teaching_tips.asp*

~

Some nonverbal children and adults cannot process visual and auditory input at the same time. They are mono-channel. They cannot see and hear at the same time. They should not be asked to look and listen at the same time. They should be given either a visual task or an auditory task. Their immature nervous system is not able to process simultaneous visual and auditory input.

> —*Temple Grandin, PhD, author of* Thinking in Pictures *and* The Way I See It; *www.autism.com/ind_teaching_tips.asp*

~

Tips for Homeschooling and Basic Skills

Contact the Home School Legal Defense Association, their website will provide information about the laws in each state, which tend to vary as to subjects required and parent qualifications.

When designing your own curriculum, check out homeschool support groups (Google) and *The World Book,* which provides an online guide (for free) detailing typical courses for each grade.

~

The following tips are adapted from "Beginning to Homeschool a Child with an Autism Spectrum Disorder" by Valorie Delp, Famlies.com, www.homeschooling.families. com/blog/7-tips-for-beginning- to-homeschool-a-child-an-autism-spectrum-disorder.

- Most experts seem to feel that the beginning of homeschooling for a child with an ASD is to "de-school." The technical definition of this would be for your child to "unlearn" all the negative socialization experiences he had in school. Many homeschooling veterans point to this as a time for you to observe your child, and for your child to really explore areas that interest him. Learning must again become fun.

- While "de-schooling," contact local organizations and support groups. Try to make contact with other parents who understand both autism and homeschooling.

- Keep a journal. You might want to consider taking notes at this time. What helps your child focus? What are his favorite things, and what is he doing when happiest? Where does he excel?

- Ditch your preconceptions. Try to approach the process with an open mind. Think about your end goal and then work backwards: What will get you to your end goal with your child? It is likely to look different than traditional schooling would be, and that's just fine!

- Determine where your child is on checklists and evaluations. Set a goal and then work toward that goal. On the other hand . . . ditch the checklist if it is too frustrating. In states where there is a lot of paperwork, you can document your child's progress toward the goal and why you stopped pursuing it.

- Locate needed therapies and services for your child. There is a variety of resources available, and with a little legwork at the library, I've heard of many parents providing needed therapy at home as appropriate.

Educational

~

Begin teaching independence and daily living skills early on. It might take your child some time to perfect them. It's better to start earlier than later. Try things like having them set the table for dinner or prepare their own lunch.

~

Even if your child cannot complete the entire task, break down daily routines to give them a role. For example, give your child a shoelace to pull when untying laces, fasten the zipper and then allow your child to finish the task by pulling the zipper up, etc. Add more steps as your child's skills develop to further increase his independence.

CHAPTER 6

Diagnosis & Doctors

Diagnosis

noun

1. the identification of the nature of an illness or other problem by examination of the symptoms: *early diagnosis and treatment are essential*

Finding Your Way

If you have any hint that your child's development is off, it should be handled at the youngest possible age, as we now know that early intervention leads to better outcomes. Bring to your pediatrician's attention any apparent delay or symptom (*see list below*), and do not accept "It's a phase" or "Don't worry" from anyone. Seek a second opinion if necessary.

Symptoms of Autism

There are many lists out there describing symptoms of autism via Google. We present a sample grouping below. Review, and if you note any delays see your pediatrician. Remember to err on the side of caution; it will help you catch any issues early when prognosis is better.

Diagnosis & Doctors

Speech Problems:

- Nonverbal (unable to speak, perhaps has a few words)
- Repetitive—repeating phrases over
- Inappropriate speech—speech which makes little sense
- Echolalia—repeating the vocalizations of another
- Scripting—repeating lines from a movie or TV show over and over

Social Problems:

- Does not understand typical social boundaries or behavior in social situations
- Decreased imaginary and pretend play
- Extremely hyperactive or underactive
- Extreme tantrums—uncontrollable
- Tunes others out, plays by self
- Frequently does not notice someone entering the room
- Inappropriate playing with toys or prefers objects that are not toys
- Poor eye contact
- Lack of fear in dangerous situations (climbing on shelves)
- Often does not return a happy smile from parents
- Difficulty with transitions (could be location or activity transitions)

<u>Sensory Problems:</u>

- Unusual pain tolerance
- Avoids close contact or makes unusually close contact (looks into face)
- Frequently annoyed by certain sensations such as clothing tags, wearing shoes, and/or avoids or seeks out certain textures (sand, carpeting, grass)
- Bothered by large noisy, crowds
- Sensory seeking—requires deep pressure squeezing, hugging, and/or massage

<u>Movement Problems:</u>

- Self-stimulating behaviors (known as "stimming"; i.e. hand flapping, repetitive movements, lining up objects)
- Self-restricted diet (eats only chicken nuggets)
- Unusually aggressive or self-injurious behaviors (head banging, bites self)
- Obsessed with routines (avoids change)
- Obsession with spinning objects

NOTE: Children who are at risk (particularly those whose parents have auto–immune conditions or siblings on the spectrum) should be watched very closely for any of the symptoms listed above.

~

KEY TIP

Labels: I don't much care for labels of any sort, but in the case of autism, don't be afraid of the label, because it will help you get the services you need. To garner the highest amount of services for your child, do not shy away from an autism diagnosis. If your son is on the border of autism and "high-functioning," go for the full autism diagnosis—you will receive more hours of therapy, and the diagnosis can always be adjusted later with improvement. Additionally, if your son is on the autism/mental retardation (MR) border, work to get the autism label—again, the level and amount of therapy is superior, given perceived better outcomes for autism over MR.

~

Once you have determined that your child's development and behavior profile contains autistic manifestations and features, you will be guided (by a variety of well-intentioned and well-meaning professionals or parents) onto the "Autism Superhighway." Do not allow yourself to journey down the road marked cure. Instead, travel down the road toward recovery. The journey to recovery will not be a sprint but a marathon. There will be times when the road is smooth and straight and times when there will be curves, dead ends, and detours. Find yourself a developmental pediatrician or another professional who is willing to be your guide and GPS system. Avoid cookie-cutter approaches, interventions, and action plans. Instead, let your child's unique and individual profile guide you on this journey.

—Dr. Mark Freilich, Total Kids
Developmental Pediatric Resources, New York City

~

Contact the local chapters of the Autism Society of America (ASA), the National Autism Association (NAA), Autism Speaks, Generation Rescue (GR), and Talk About Curing Autism (TACA), and find parents to connect with and learn from. They can share information about doctors and diagnoses (and schools and more). Professionals are often restricted when it comes to the information they can share.

Finding Doctors & Dentists

The parent network route is the best way to find the doctors and dentists who are most experienced and friendly to the autism community. As mentioned previously, you can join one or more of the many organizations mentioned in this book (NAA, GR, TACA, etc.) all of which have excellent networking options to find doctors and dentists. In addition, parents in support groups or via your child's school are another good source. You can also look at the websites for NAA, GR, TACA, ARI (Autism Research

Institute) and the Medical Academy of Pediatric Special
Needs (or MAPS, www.medmaps.org/clinician-directory/)
all have lists of doctors in your area.

~

Here are some questions to ask when choosing a doctor for
your child:

- Approximately how many individuals with autism have
  you treated? What age range?
- In the event we have a biomedical-related emergency,
  how will I contact you?
- Do you share an e-mail address, cellphone number, etc.
  with your patients?
- Can you collaborate with other specialists we will be
  dealing with (gastrointestinal, etc.)? Are you willing to
  collaborate on treatment and testing with my child's
  pediatrician if he or she is receptive?
- Will you provide a clear plan for supplements and
  where to purchase them?
- What are the primary medical specialties in which you
  were originally trained (i.e., pediatrics, family medicine)?
  What is now the primary focus of your practice? If you
  are not an MD or DO, in what field(s) are you licensed?
- Do you sell proprietary nutritional supplements or have
  a sales agreement with supplement suppliers? Do you
  sell supplements at cost?

- Do you bill for laboratory tests done by commercial laboratories? How do you break down the fees?

—Autism Research Institute,
www.autism.com/treating_finding

~

Make sure your child's doctor is one whom you are comfortable with, and who specializes in treating the medical needs of kids with autism. He or she should be regularly attending autism medical conferences to keep up-to-date, and ideally be someone who regularly communicates with other autism experts. Parents must educate themselves and exercise caution when selecting a clinician.

~

When looking for a dentist for your ASD child, search for those who specialize in ASD kids. If you do not have one of these specialists nearby focus on pediatric dentists, as they will be more than likely to have been exposed to special-needs kids and be better equipped to handle them. Some might even have a specific day of the week when they only schedule kids with special needs. Also don't neglect the all-important parent network, and ask the parents of your child's classmates for references.

Dental Tips

From Ruby Gelman, DMD, New York City

- I have found that short, more frequent visits prove to be very successful in the dental office. I will recommend seeing autistic kids every two to four months, and at each visit, we do the same things we did at the visit before, while incorporating something new each time. Kids will remember things better from one visit to the next.

- Be sure to choose a dentist who has experience treating kids who are on the autistic spectrum. The experienced dentist will be happy to speak to you prior to the appointment to formulate an appropriate treatment approach.

- While many dentists recommend sedation for autistic kids, I do not believe it is appropriate if this is suggested without meeting your child in the dental office setting first.

- If your child has an object that he particularly loves (a music player or clock, for example), bring one with you to the dental visit so that the dentist can incorporate that into the appointment.

~

Pretending to be examined yourself may help ease the anxiety your child feels upon doctor or dental visits. If the doctor/dentist agrees, you may be able to interest your child in some of the equipment in the office; many kids enjoy riding up and down on the examination chair or running it themselves.

And Regarding Dental Hygene from Dr. Gelman:

- Be persistent with tooth brushing, even if it is difficult. Be sure to make brushing teeth a routine part of your child's routine, morning and night. Start by counting to ten slowly while brushing so that your child knows when it will be over. Gradually add more time so that you are able to brush the entire mouth well.

- Water is a great help to keep the mouth clean after meals. Drinking a few ounces of water after a meal can significantly reduce the acid buildup that begins with chewing and swallowing food. This can be a great help in preventing cavities.

- Not every toothbrush is acceptable. For example, try different kinds of toothbrushes with softer bristles, a different-shaped head, or different textured bristles, or different flavors of toothpaste or gels. We have had success with Oral B's battery-powered line.

- Different brushing techniques should also be tried to avoid various sensations, and saliva levels in the mouth should be carefully monitored.

~

NOTE: On June 12, 2008, the FDA admitted on its website that silver fillings in our teeth are toxic and harmful to our health, and that they "might have neuro-toxic effects on the nervous systems of developing children and fetuses." Avoid them. Likewise, research fluoride before allowing fluoride treatments or using fluoride toothpaste. If you have them (silver fillings) yourself, you can get them removed with the help of insurance.

CHAPTER 7

Safety

A Spectrum of Concerns

This is the most important chapter in the book. Safety from wandering (49 percent of all kids with autism wander at some point), from abuse, from navigating the neighborhood; parents with kids on the spectrum have many safety concerns. My son has wandered himself, and was gone for more than two hours on one occasion, in New York City no less. I start this chapter with a description of that event and then introduce Tips to help with wandering and other safety concerns. At the end of this chapter I am including a section on Managing Wandering by Lori McIlwain of the National Autism Association, which is known for their safety programs.

~

September 2, 2013—Manhattan, Upper East Side
So my son ran today. More of a stroll really, but I guess the official term is "run." I've written before on my blog about how he has "escaped" from my apartment

here in NYC, and typically been found by neighbors in the building and or the doormen. Today was different.

I had a sitter here working with Alex; I was out riding my bike in Central Park. When I returned home, my doorman told me Alex was missing and the staff was looking for him. This has happened before, however when he told me how Alex had been gone, for over thirty minutes, I felt sick. That was new. His adventures before lasted about five minutes or so, before cameras or residents found him. I should say he is quite noisy and tough to miss. Most in our neighborhood know him on sight, luckily (a good reason to stay put I guess).

Upon learning Alex was gone for such a long time, I quickly joined the hunt. Our high-rise is connected to a smaller building via a stairwell. This smaller "back" building houses mostly retired folks, who in the past have contacted the front desk upon finding Alex wandering their halls (overall, this has happened maybe four times). This time he was spotted getting on an elevator (separate elevators for the two buildings). As I searched, I learned he had been spotted there and focused on the "back" building. Staff was in both buildings (along with some fellow residents and Alex's worried sitter) climbing stairwells, riding elevators, and checking roofs, back gardens, the street. I ran around the outside of the building, asking dog walkers, doormen, garage attendants, and random passersby if Alex had been spotted. Again, Alex as a fifteen-year-old curly blonde–haired, noisy yet non-verbal boy is tough to miss. After about an hour, or I should say an HOUR, the front desk of the building got me on my cell and said the police had brought Alex in.

What had happened was that Alex had gotten out through the "back" building to the street and decided to walk towards 2nd Avenue (we live on 3rd) and a kindly neighbor in another apartment building realized something was up and actually knew of Alex (just from being in the neighborhood) and took him in (she has a townhome). After giving him a sandwich and banana, she called the police, and they jointly returned him to our building. Police suggest a bracelet with the usual "lost" information, however Alex can easily rip that off (and has). My best bet is to add an inside lock and key. Needless to say it was quite the way to end Labor Day Weekend.

My purpose in sharing this is twofold. One, to just help me unwind! The other, to communicate to those who have experienced similar "runs" that they are not alone, and that people, our neighbors, the police can be caring and concerned. Some of the neighbors and police officers involved hugged and slapped my back in a show of support. I thank them all!

Running Tips

The following tips are adapted from Autistic Spectrum Disorders: Understanding the Diagnosis & Getting Help *by Mitzi Waltz.*

Published by O'Reilly Media, Inc. Copyright © 2002 Mitzi Waltz. All rights reserved. Used with permission. www.oreilly.com/medical/autism/news/tips_life.html

If escapes are a problem for your family, please consider using the services of a professional security consultant. You may be able to get help from government developmental-delay or mental health agencies, or private agencies, to find and even pay for these services. Most people don't wish to turn their homes into fortresses, but in some cases, it's the most caring thing you can do. It could very well save a life.

~

Double- or triple-bolt security doors can slow down a would-be escapee, and some types can be unlocked only from the inside with a key. While expensive, they are tremendously jimmy-proof. Keep the keys well hidden, of course—on your person, if need be. Fire regulations may require that an exterior-lock key be secured in a firebox or stored at the nearest fire station in case of emergency.

Bars can also be placed on windows, as many homeowners in urban areas already do. Like key locks, these can be a fire hazard. A security consultant, or perhaps your local fire department, may be able to come up with ideas. Some types of bars have interior latches.

Alarms are available that will warn you if a nocturnal roamer is approaching a door or window. Other types only sound when the door or window is actually opened. Depending on your child's speed, the latter may not give you enough response time.

Obviously, fences and gates are a good idea for backyards. Some types are less easily scaled than others. Although it might seem cruel, in extreme cases a child's safety could be secured by using electric fencing (usually this involves a single "live" wire at the top of a tall fence). Electric fencing kits are available at some hardware stores or at farm-supply stores.

For gates, key locks are more secure than latches.

Electronic locks of various types are another option, including remote control and keypad varieties. These can be used for garage doors, gates, or exterior doors.

~

Help from Law Enforcement

In some cities, local police departments are sensitive to the needs and special problems of the disabled. Officers may be available to provide information about keeping your child or adult patient safe and secure, whether he lives in your home, in an institution or group home, or independently in the community. Some also have special classes to teach self-defense skills to disabled adults.

A few police departments also keep a registry of disabled people whose behavior could be a hazard to their own safety, or whose behavior could be misinterpreted as threatening. Avail yourself of this service if your child is an escape artist, has behaviors that could look like drunkenness or drug use to an uninformed observer, uses threatening words or gestures when afraid, or is extremely trusting of strangers.

~

Take the time to inform your local law enforcement agency and emergency personnel that a child with special needs resides at your home and may require special attention during an emergency.

As with the tip above, inform your neighbors about your special needs child, especially if he is a runner. Providing photos and contact information can be a lifesaver. I have photos of Alex with contact information printed on the back.

Personal Identification (ID) Options

People with ASDs can have a bracelet or necklace made with their home phone number, an emergency medical contact number, or the phone number of a service that can inform the caller about their diagnosis. Labels you might want to have engraved on this item include:

- Nonverbal
- Speech-impaired
- Multiple medications
- Medications include . . . (list)
- Epilepsy (or other medical condition)

Members of the general public, and even some safety officials, may not know the word "autistic." They are even more unlikely to know what autistic spectrum disorder (ASD) or pervasive developmental disorder (PDD) means.

~

There are incredible programs out there like Project Lifesaver (www.ProjectLifesaver.org). Project Lifesaver has been commonly used with Alzheimer's patients, but has grown to address the needs of others, including those with autism, Down syndrome, traumatic brain injury, and more. People who qualify for the program are given a tracking device with a unique frequency to wear as a bracelet, which emergency responders can pick up and track with specialized equipment from one to several miles away. If your child has already gotten away from you—at home or in a public place—or you are afraid they will, see if there's a Project Lifesaver in your community and contact them.

They do amazing work. There's almost always a wait list, so get on it if you qualify.

—*Tim Tucker, "Practical Ideas for Protecting Autistic Children Before they Disappear," www.bothhandsandaflashlight. com/2010/04/16/practical-ideas-for-protecting-autistic-children-before-they-disappear*

~

Start by choosing a comfortable sport-band style ID or a silicone wristband in your child's favorite color, personalized with your name and emergency contact information. Persist as much as possible to encourage your little runner to keep it on. (Is the wrist simply a no-go? Try his ankle.) Another option is to use iron-on labels on his clothes.

—*Mary Fetzer, "Keeping Your Autistic Child Safe,"* She Knows, *Home & Garden*

~

There are permanent ink stamps for kids' clothing if tags or bracelets create sensory issues. Placing on the outside is advisable for viewing, and these items are totally unobtrusive to your child's sensory needs. These labels can be customized with name, contact information and specifics, such as non-verbal.

~

For Alex we now have something called RoadID (www.
roadid.com), which was designed for runners in remote
locations, but works great as an ID tag for wandering
autistic kids. Check out the site and note the ID's are
unobtrusively placed on shoes and can contain descriptive
information along with ID.

Preventing & Preparing for Wandering

Know the signs. Your best defense against something terrible
happening is to notice patterns in your child's behavior that
might indicate they are about to try to escape or otherwise
take off in a way that could put them in serious danger,
such as running off a sidewalk into a street. Noticing any
strong interests, especially ones that get more intense, might
help in knowing when and where they might wander off to
fulfill those interests.

*—Tim Tucker, "Practical Ideas for Protecting Autistic
Children Before they Disappear," www.bothhandsandaflashlight.
com/2010/04/16/practical-ideas-for-protecting-autistic-
children-before-they-disappear*

~

Visual symbols of stop signs or other such signage can be
used in the home and are easily purchased on the Internet.
Google "street signs" and you'll find plenty of options.
These symbols can stall a child from taking flight.

~

Using an alarm system, dead bolts, and window locks are necessary to secure your residence, especially if your kid is a runner.

~

As with infants, a speaker system or even a video monitor can serve to provide a level of comfort and help you transition a child into his/her own room.

~

Key is to avert your child from getting outside to begin with. A good strategy is to create several layers of "defense" against flight. This way, if total prevention from bolting is unreasonable, you can at least slow them down and buy time for your pursuit or search. For instance, you can set up things that will keep him in a particular area or warn if he escapes outside said area. So gates in various parts of the home that may be opened but that are alarmed or provide some visual or auditory feedback to the parent/caregiver can do the job. Likewise door chimes & motion detectors can cover doors and windows. Google these items; there are versions that are inexpensive and these items can be reimbursed with a Medicaid waiver.

~

Set up "outdoor traps" in your yard or outside your apartment. I wish I could take credit for this idea, as it's brilliant. Here's where you can leverage your child's intense interests to great advantage. This particular parent's child loves pinwheels, so she put pinwheels on various objects and in the ground in strategic places in her yard. One time he got out, but he saw one of the pinwheels and just stood there playing with it rather than continuing to run. It bought her the minute or two she needed to find him and stop him from going any farther. Figure out how to take your child's interests and convert them into a system that will at least stall them or keep them from going any farther.

—*Tim Tucker, "Practical Ideas for Protecting Autistic Children Before they Disappear," www.bothhandsandaflashlight. com/2010/04/16/practical-ideas-for-protecting-autistic-children-before-they-disappear*

~

A smart phone, tablet or other device can serve to aid as in tracking down a runner. Learn to use the GPS function. Enable the "find device" option on your child's device and check periodically from a computer.

~

If you have a runner, know where in your neighborhood your child gravitates. These will be the likely destinations.

You can also increase your frequency of visits to these locations to lessen the fascination with them.

~

Swimming is not only a great exercise for your child, but can serve as a safety tool as well. Frequently, kids with autism favor water and water-based activities. Keep your kid safe with some lessons.

Personal Safety

Teaching the concept of "private" to little boys will help them understand important rules of private vs. public behavior. As they get older, it's important to have additional conversations about the topic, to help them understand rules of personal safety. At home, teach your son that it is okay to have clothes off in private areas of the house (i.e., their bedroom), but that in public areas of the house (living room, kitchen, etc.), they must keep their clothes on. Use picture icons if needed.

~

Relationship boundaries are difficult concepts for boys on the spectrum and must be taught and practiced. First, your boy needs to learn about different types of relationships (i.e., husband, wife, close friend, colleague, neighbor, shopkeeper). Then, he needs to be taught the concept of appropriate types of conversations and behaviors for the different relationships.

~

Boys on the spectrum need to know what constitutes sexual abuse. Nonverbal children and teens are at a high risk for sexual and physical abuse because of the perception that they are unable to communicate what happens to them. They are often grouped in classrooms or camp situations where predators know they can find victims.

Boys on the more able end of the spectrum are also at high risk for sexual abuse because they are not good at figuring out people's intentions (i.e., picking up on nonverbal cues). This is why it's important for them to be taught what constitutes a sexual act and what is appropriate and inappropriate behavior.

It is important for the boy's safety that he be able to identify places on his body where it is inappropriate to be touched by others. It is important that the boy be able to communicate to someone when he has been touched in an "off-limits" area on his body. Off-limits areas of the body are those normally covered by a bathing suit. Additionally, best not to tell a child on the autism spectrum to always obey grown-ups.

Car Safety

Especially for younger kids, escaping from their car seat can be one of the worst problems we encounter. For kids still in the five-point harness, you can simply take the lap part that everything buckles into and flip it over such that the button is facing down into the child's lap. For other kids, especially those using the regular seat belt, there are covers available that make it difficult for them to get to that release button.

Always enable the child locks on the rear doors of your vehicle. If adult passengers riding in your backseat complain, tell them they can walk home.

~

Local chapters of National Autism Association, Autism Society, and others have stickers available to members that can be put on a car window. This lets emergency responders know that your child is autistic and might not respond to verbal instructions.

Toxin Removal from Home and Diet

More and more, it is becoming recognized that many of the symptoms of autism are related to environmental toxins. Working on repairing any toxic burden can lead to better outcomes and better health for our children and selves. Following are some tips to help remove potential sources of toxins in the household.

~

The following tips are adapted from the article "Emerging Science Combined with Common Sense Gives Parents Better Options for

Preventing Autism" by Maureen McDonnell, RN, The Autism File*, Issue 35, 2010.*

- Switch to green cleaning and personal-care products (e.g., shampoo, toothpaste, body lotion, facial cream). The average American home contains three to ten gallons of hazardous materials, and 85 percent of the chemicals that are registered have never been tested for their impact on the human body. See the Green This! series of books by Deirdre Imus.

- Eat organically grown grains, vegetables, fruits, nuts, meat, chicken, and eggs.

- If a woman has taken many drugs—prescription or over-the-counter—or works or lives in a chemically laden environment, she might consider a detoxification or cleansing program.

- Find a "green" dry cleaner (the chemical used in most dry-cleaning facilities, perchlorethylene, is a known carcinogen).

- Use a stainless-steel water bottle to carry and consume filtered water. Heated or not, the soft plastic bottles will release phthalates. Antimony can also be released from polyethylene terephthalate.

- For more information about water filters, call 1-800-673-8010 or visit NSF International's website, at www. nsf.org/ Certified/DWTU/ and the Natural Resources

Defense Council website at www.nrdc.org/water/drinking/gfilters.asp.

- Safely remove mercury-based amalgam fillings with a dentist associated with the American Holistic Dental Association (www.holisticdental.org) at least six months before becoming pregnant, and not while breastfeeding.

- Prior to conceiving, consult a natural health-care clinician or physician well versed in treating GI disturbances, as well as elevated levels of toxins and heavy metals. One option is to contact a naturopathic physician (ND) or an MD associated with the American College for Advancement in Medicine (www.acamnet.org).

~

When painting, choose low- or no-VOC (volatile organic compounds) paints. Select green building or remodeling products and allow adequate time for "non-green" building materials to outgas before moving back into the newly built or renovated nursery, room, or home. Reduce exposure to electromagnetic radiation by eliminating the use of microwave ovens, keeping cell-phone usage to a minimum, and storing your cell phone in your bag rather than in your pocket.

~

Minimize consumption of large fish (for mercury levels of fish, check www.gotmercury.org for a mercury in fish calculator). In general, avoid large fish, which have the highest concentrations of mercury; focus on freshwater species.

~

To build beneficial microflora, take high-quality probiotics (in addition to improving levels of beneficial intestinal flora, these have been shown to decrease intestinal absorption of certain chemicals by facilitating their excretion) and consume more fermented foods. Try adding organic sauerkraut to spaghetti squash for example.

More Quick Household Tips

- Do not sleep near a computer or other wireless device.
- Improve indoor air quality by opening the windows and creating cross ventilation.
- Use natural methods for controlling household and garden pests.
- Have children avoid playing on pressure-treated wood decks and swing sets (source of arsenic).
- Minimize the use of fire-retardant sleepwear (contains the toxic material antimony).
- Purchase organic mattresses and linens.

- Remove shoes before entering the home to prevent contaminants from soil coming into the house.
- Choose foods that are less processed and clean of chemicals and toxins. Why? Because children with autism are already compromised nutritionally. Use organic options whenever possible.
- Tap water should be avoided, as it contains many different kinds of contaminants; invest in a good filtration system.
- Check your home for toxins such as lead and mold.
- If you have a fireplace, avoid burning treated wood.

Managing Wandering Tendencies in Children & Adults with Autism

By Lori McIlwain, National Autism Association

At the National Autism Association, we often hear from fellow parents who worry about their child or adult wandering away from home or school. With 49% of children with autism prone to going missing according to a 2012 *Pediatrics* study, coupled with stories of children drowning, it's natural for us to feel some level of anxiety.

The good news is that more awareness creates more tools, and prevention resources. What was once absent is now beginning to crop up among nonprofit organizations, government agencies, and medical establishments. Even so, parents continue to seek new ways to protect their children, and because search time is limited, *a multi-layered approach is key.*

A multi-layered approach simply means having several levels of protection as opposed to relying on one solution. Because every child/adult with autism is different, custom safeguards are likely necessary. That said, the data we've been able to collect over the years has captured a few clues as to what could help us prevent—and respond to—a wandering incident.

Self-Protection

Easier said than done, but self-protection is the first line of defense, and helping a child understand ways to keep themselves safe is the ultimate goal. Many parents implement progress protocols centered on therapies, medical needs, treating underlying conditions, and creating a behavioral intervention plan. Because wandering behaviors are a form of communication (i.e., I want, I need, I don't want, etc.), communication aids are a great safety tool for both verbal and nonverbal children, as are social stories & schedules. Be sure to identify and address the reason behind the behaviors, and use motivators and repetition to build safety skills. Find social stories at awaare.org.

Supervision

Supervision is essential, but hyper-vigilance is especially critical during times of commotion, after a new move, during vacations, holidays, warmer weather, outdoor activities, school and other transitions. Be careful not to assume more eyes equals more protection. Many parents use the "tag" system during holiday parties and other high-commotion times. This is a simple approach of assigning one responsible adult to be your child's primary supervisor during an agreed-upon period of time. Make sure the tagged caregiver understands his/her responsibilities and expectations.

TIP: School supervision should not be loosened for the sake of teaching independence. If your child's school insists on teaching independence before your child is ready, re-direct them to the concept of pre-independence, which entails an "eyes on, hands off" way of teaching safety skills, danger awareness, self-help skills, self-regulation and survival skills—all of which can naturally lead to a safe form of

*independence. Written and agreed-upon plans should be
created in an organized, thoughtful and consistent manner
that begins with understanding your child and bases safe
teaching methods on how your child will best respond.*

Security

Basic security includes adequate locks, such as
deadbolt and hook-and-eye locks, but other essentials
include door alarms, stop signs on doors/windows,
fencing, and avoiding the use of window A/C units,
fans or screens. Some parents also use baby monitors
and home security systems. Keep garage door openers
out of reach, and if you own a pool, it is imperative
that you put a fence around it. Use gates that self-
close and self-latch higher than your children's reach.
Remember to remove all pool toys when not in use.

*TIP: Visit BigRedSafetyShop.com or Radio Shack for
GE door/window alarms, affordable enough to buy for hotel
rooms and other non-home settings.*

Survival Skills

When a child with autism wanders off, the most
immediate threats include water, traffic and

encounters with strangers or police. Swimming lessons are critical. Find an autism-friendly YMCA by visiting nationalautismassociation.org or ask your pediatrician if there are organizations that offer swimming lessons for children with special needs in your area. Some of your child's swim lessons should include lessons with his/her clothes and shoes on. Also teach name, address, and phone number using whatever means possible, and always have an ID on your child.

TIP: Sound reduction/cancellation earmuffs can help reduce stress or triggers. You can find brands like Peltor at Lowes, Home Depot, or online at Amazon.com.

Safeguards

Safeguards may include tracking devices, distance monitors, wearable ID bracelets (we like RoadID.com) and ID cards. If you need a short-term solution, temporary tattoos are a great option. For tracking devices, check out projectlifesaver.org, lojacksafetynet.com, or iloctech.com. My Buddy Tags and Angel Alert Distance Monitors make a nice secondary safeguard for public outings. For nighttime wanderers, especially teens and adults, use a pajama shirt to alert bystanders like the ones found at BigRedSafetyShop. com.

Search-and-Rescue

If your child is ever missing, stay calm, call 911, and search areas that pose the most immediate threats, such as water and traffic. Even those children/adults who demonstrate a fear or dislike of water may perceive lakes, ponds and rivers quite differently. Varying colors, reflective patterns and other factors may tempt curiosity, so do not disregard nearby water sources as a possible location for your missing child. Neighbors and first responders can be your child's life-line in the event of an emergency, so prepare them ahead of time. Provide essential information about your child, nearby water sources, favorite attractions, medical information, emergency contact information and other relevant details. Download and prepare a family wandering emergency plan by visiting awaare.org.

Bolting: A Category all its Own

While wandering behaviors are typically a form of communication, bolting can have the added elements of impulsivity and unpredictability. It can be a type of trigger that sets a child or adult in motion—a noise, a fear, a desire. The abruptness and speed of bolting makes it especially dangerous, particularly in open public environments.

If your child tends to bolt, ask his/her school for a functional behavioral assessment. Based on its findings, a behavioral intervention plan should be developed and used consistently between home and school. If you're going out in a public place, communicate safety rules beforehand. Use a picture schedule or social story to help your child understand expectations. Walking arm-in-arm helps prevent bolting incidents in areas like a parking lot. For walking or hiking, use a bookends approach with one adult on each side of the child.

A school 1:1 should be assigned to any child or teen with autism at risk of bolting or wandering off, but the use of restraints should never be encouraged as they may have a lasting negative effect. Non-emergency restraint, prone or supine restraints, and seclusion practices could cause new behaviors or worsen existing ones. Reducing or eliminating triggers while creating ways for your child to deescalate will help prevent bolting incidents and the need for emergency restraint.

A multi-layered approach is critical in preventing and addressing a wandering incident. Ideally, underlying causes of wandering behaviors should be identified and addressed. Remember, the ultimate goal is for children to understand potential dangers and to learn ways to keep themselves safe.

To learn more, visit awaare.org. For help with strategies, write to lori@nationalautism.org. For those at extreme risk, contact Kennedy Krieger Institute at (443) 923-9400.

CHAPTER 8
Puberty

It is the sandstorm that shapes the stone statues of the desert. It is the struggles of life that form a person's character.

—Native American Proverb

The Best of Times, The Worst of Times

Many parents dread the approach of puberty for multiple reasons. Frequently challenging behaviors increase, albeit temporarily, as hormonal changes kick in, creating anxiety in our kids. Extra patience during this period is advisable (see chapter on Self-Care, which I told you not to skip!). As Alex is now beyond sixteen, I have noticed improvements coming out of this time, so hold on, things get better.

In addition there are concerns about the changes themselves and appropriate behavior in regards to. Below I provide some tips from my experience and that of others, which have been helpful.

Discussing Puberty

Boys who do not like change may get upset when they see their body beginning to change and grow differently, and they realize they have no control over it. Explaining that everyone's body changes, and showing baby, children, teen, and current photos of adult family members will help them understand that puberty and growing happens to everyone.

Also, make sure to use correct names of body parts (i.e., penis, vagina), but also teach the synonyms that they may hear from others (i.e., boobs).

~

Explain that some changes will only be associated with the same sex (e.g., a boy will not begin to grow breasts, but a girl will). Explain that hair will only grow in certain places (the child may think the whole body eventually becomes progressively covered in hair, like a werewolf). Explain that extra hair just grows on the underarms and on the pubic area in women. Explain that on men, extra hair grows on the underarms and on the pubic area, and on the chest, face, and chin.

~

It is important to begin teaching boys about their changing bodies before they hit puberty. Teaching them about the changes that will occur in the girl's body as well as their own body is important. Otherwise, they may be surprised by the changes they see in their female classmates, and not understand why they look different if they have not seen them for some time (i.e., summer vacation).

~

To prevent teenage boys from giving the wrong "signal," teach them that staring at certain parts of another's anatomy is rude and inappropriate. The rule should be that a person should never stare at the private parts of another person's body, the area normally covered by a bathing suit (male or female). An ASD teen boy may not be able to "read" the cues from another person as to whether the interest is reciprocal. The teen needs to have explicit instruction about indications that someone likes them, as opposed to being interested romantically.

Masturbation Issues

Masturbation is normal teenage activity; however, most teenagers know to masturbate in private. Not so for boys on the spectrum. Parents need to teach their teenage boys the concept of private and public, and that masturbation is a private activity, not a public one.

~

If a teenage boy is attempting to masturbate at school, the best thing to do is redirect. At home, teens should be allowed a private place (their bedroom) to masturbate, and should be redirected there if they attempt to masturbate elsewhere in the house.

~

Touching in the genital area should be addressed as soon as noticed regardless of age. Just say matter-of-factly: "Touching your penis is for private time. Please wait till you are in bed or in the bedroom." There is no room for emotions here. If you are vague or nervous, your child will likely continue to grow more inappropriate. Be clear and nonjudgmental. It has worked well for us.

Behavior Changes During Puberty

When boys reach puberty and start showing more noncompliant behaviors, many parents think "Oh no—his autism is getting worse!" Actually, noncompliance is normal teenage behavior. At this point, parents need to remember to give the teen more choices in which to express himself and to have more control over some aspects of his day, within defined limits.

~

Precocious puberty has been estimated to be twenty times higher in children with neurodevelopmental disabilities, including autism.

~

In my case, the anxiety seized me for no good reason. Many people with autism find that the symptoms worsen at puberty. When my anxiety went away, it was replaced with bouts of colitis or terrible headaches. My nervous system was constantly under stress.

—*Temple Grandin, PhD,* Thinking in Pictures

~

Puberty can be a difficult time for a boy on the spectrum, as usually they like predictability and routine, and many have a difficult time with change. Many have a hard time with the fact that their body is growing and changing and there is nothing they can do to stop it.

Sexual Educational Tips

From Dr. Mary Jo Lang, Beacon Day School

- Don't be afraid to address sexuality and sexual behavior with children and adolescents who have autism, as they have the same basic human needs like everyone else. Failure to address this subject matter can lead to confusion, inappropriate behavior, and/or things that can be both physically and emotionally damaging. Start educating children with autism about their sexuality early on. It is most beneficial when the information comes from their parent/caregiver.

- Reassure the child/adolescent that these feelings and desires are common, and it's okay to be experiencing them. Encourage them to ask questions and not to be embarrassed.

- Determine your comfort level in discussing sexuality and sex with your teenage son. Look for resources and specialists if you feel it would be helpful to you. Determine where your boy is at in his development. Obtain social and emotional age-appropriate materials to use while teaching him what he needs to know.

- If the teenage boy is physically mature but delayed socially and emotionally, but is also gregarious, communicate openly and consistently with the boy's teachers, care providers, and, if appropriate, with local authorities, on where the boy is at in development, as well as what you are teaching them. This will help prevent social and/or legal issues arising from any possible inappropriate public behavior.

- Teach your son early and often the basics about sexual awareness: What is sex, what is acceptable behavior, and when is it acceptable? Teach about boundaries: What boundaries should we have for our bodies, as well as when interacting with others?

- Hypersensitivity or hyposensitivity due to sensory processing challenges may affect how a man with autism handles sexual intimacy. Extreme sensitivity may make it difficult for some young men to enjoy the physical aspects of a close relationship.

- If your son sits in on sex education classes offered at the school for the mainstream population, he may hear all the facts but not personalize the information and realize that it is meant for him. This means that as a parent, you will need to verify that he has understood how this information relates to him.

- Children and adolescents with autism tend to interpret things literally. Be clear and direct when discussing sexuality. Obtain materials that are socially and emotionally age-appropriate as well as anatomically correct when teaching your child/adolescent about sexuality and sexual behavior. Discuss the following topics with your child/adolescent: puberty, body parts, personal care, medical examination, social skills, and responsibilities surrounding sexual behavior.

- Address self-protection skills that encourage children and adolescents with autism to say "no" and to avoid individuals who seek to take advantage of them. It has been reported that children with disabilities are 2.2 times more likely to be sexually abused, making self-protection skills important to address and develop.

CHAPTER 9
Day-to-Day Life

The secret of life, though, is to fall seven times and get up
eight times.

—*Paulo Coelho*

The Daily Grind

From surviving meltdowns to toilet training to eating out,
this chapter focuses on those day-to-day trials that only
a special needs parent can understand. My goal here is to
provide practical tips for tasks and events that occur on a
regular basis, but for those of us with kids on the spectrum
are challenging and frustrating and thus debilitating due to
their recurring nature. Let's start with meltdowns.

Responding to Undesirable Behavior,
a.k.a. Meltdown Help!

A "tantrum" or "meltdown" is actually a call for help, a cry
to notice that the stress level has overflowed its container.
A word of caution to family members: Try to identify what
pushed your son beyond endurance—and don't expect
it to always be the same thing. It could be noise in high-

ceilinged supermarkets, or maybe it was the crowds, or smells, or any combination of these things. Always trust that there is a precipitating cause.

That said, just because your child has autism is no reason to steer clear of consequences for bad behavior. As with any child, he will smell weakness and take advantage if you let him get away with misbehavior.

～

Don't threaten a punishment you're not prepared to enforce. If you're not really going to cancel the birthday party, don't say you will. Don't count to three, or ten—your child will learn that he always has that long, and you didn't mean it the first time. If you teach a two-year-old, gently, but firmly, that you mean what you say, you don't have to keep teaching it—at sixteen, he will still know that you meant it the first time. Too often parents allow their children to push them around because they want to be liked, but your child will neither like nor respect you. Children crave boundaries.

～

Keep your behaviors in check. We are all prone to overreaction on occasion and these potentially intense outbursts (either positive or negative) can confuse and dysregulate your son. Keeping an even keel should be your focus.

Practice deep breathing to help you stay calm during stressful times with your child. The calmer you are, the safer your child will feel, which can help prevent meltdowns from escalating even more. This is just one of the reasons for the focus on meditation and peace of mind in chapter two. Frequently meltdowns are made worse or exacerbated by the reaction from the caregiver; it's most important not to fuel the fire.

~

Set up a safe, small, quiet space that your child can use during times of frustration and anger. This gives them a comforting place of their own where they can retreat when they need a break. Likewise, when your boy is having a meltdown, try to remove others from the situation before trying to move the dysregulated child. It could help prevent the situation from escalating.

~

Dealing with emotions is one of the more difficult areas for kids on the spectrum. One strategy you can follow is when your child gets emotional remember to "label" the emotion for him or her. Giving them a description of how they are feeling will help them to understand, learn, and manage their feelings. This can be particularly useful in battling tantrums; just remember to work on the feelings after the child has calmed. You can use PECS or other visuals to describe the emotions if the child is non-verbal. There are various apps to help with this if your child has an iPad. Also, the communications apps typically include images matched to words in feeling categories.

~

Ice: When battling the meltdown from hell, deploy ice. Chewing and holding ice can help calm your son down. He can also help in the creation and storage of ice in the freezer, giving him a reference point. Many boys will seek out a particular sensory input when on the verge of melting down; ice can serve as one more tool to help them self regulate. So remember, when in hell, freeze it over!

~

KEY TIP

Parents who are dealing with their autistic child's problematic behaviors are encouraged to examine how they might be reinforcing them. For instance, the parents of an autistic child who tends to throw screaming tantrums throughout the day might be trying to put his tantrums on extinction. The parents might be successfully ignoring the tantrums while at home, but when he throws a tantrum at the playground, his parents might pick him up and bring him home to avoid creating a scene. Being picked up and carried home from the playground may in fact be reinforcing to the child, and therefore increase the likelihood that the tantrum behavior will continue.

—*Jennifer Clark, "Applied Behavior Analysis,"*
Cutting-Edge Therapies for Autism

~

Parents should work with schools in this regard, too; some children use this behavior as a way to get out of class or sent home, and if the school removes them, it just shows them they can get their way.

So communicate daily with your son's teacher or other school contacts to assess how behavior changes for the good or bad when in and out of school. He might be more regulated at school because of greater sensory opportunities via a swing or other OT equipment. You might be able to copy some, or remove other items that are helping or hindering.

~

When you sense a tantrum developing, shift gears and work to redirect your child's focus. Keep handy chewy toys, ice, or a favorite video, which may help nip a meltdown in the bud. Teach all your child's caregivers the warning signs and share strategies with them and other parents.

~

Ignore the tantrum. Seriously—this can work. Of course, it can only be applied at home. You could ignore a tantrum once you've brought him home from an off-site meltdown. A frustration meltdown has the best synergy with this strategy, as he will likely move on to something else, or just run out of steam. Then you can follow up with some queries as to what happened and try to understand what you can do to avoid this next time.

Again, keep an even keel. I know, easier said than done. But our kids are going to feed off our energy, good or bad, so work each day to keep it positive. Positive thinking may sound corny, but it does work and builds upon itself.

~

During meltdowns, work to keep everybody safe. At home you can have some strategies in place. When out in the community, this can become difficult and potentially drag others into it; it's best to remove your child from the location as quickly as possible.

~

Tantrums may scare you in their intensity, but they are typically a cry for help or understanding or even pain. It is a communication issue and your child is as afraid as you.

~

During the tantrum, offer support and comforting soothing words and actions. Do not however accede to demands made in the heat of the tantrum; it will only encourage further skirmishes.

~

I have already mentioned (multiple times) the importance of keeping a journal or diary and provided a sample worksheet (see Key Tip on page 29) to do so. Here is another use for said log—analyzing the meltdown. If you note diet, time of year, day, weather, and such in this log and track meltdowns, you may uncover a pattern that can be broken or at least properly prepared for. In my case I was able to determine that allergy season in September and April, alongside constipation, would set Alex off. I am able to preempt many a meltdown with this knowledge.

Managing Severe Aggression

Tips by Cathy Purple Cherry, AIA, LEED AP

Our ASD son was physically aggressive from the age of fourteen through now at the age of nineteen. His aggression was mostly displayed passively and through self-mutilation. On occasion, it was quite violent and sometimes directed towards his siblings. He has put his head and foot through a wall several times and punched himself to create blood and then bled all over the floor. Most recently, he attempted to stab himself with a big stick. My tips come from these past five years.

- The hardest lesson I had to teach myself was that an audience made the aggressive behavior of our ASD child worse. So, I learned to walk away, close the door, turn off the light and ignore. It took me at least three years to get to this place.

- Prevention is possible in some cases especially when it comes to reducing conflict between the ASD child and their siblings. Violation of personal space is a major trigger. Thus, prevent path crossing and entering of others' rooms. I would even orchestrate the best direction of travel around furniture to avoid conflicts.

- My son was famous for full body dropping as a negative and passive aggressive response. After he had self-mutilated, he would drop and shut down with no response whatsoever. If he was not in his own bedroom and, if I could, I removed him from our home and placed him on the grass in the yard. I watched from inside the house but absolutely did not let him know I was watching. Autistic children need time to learn to overcome their "fight" response.

- Medication changes can, at times, help. Do not hide these behaviors from your support team. Communicate immediately with your child's psychiatrist. Also, be aware that there is a calming medication that can be given just before these explosive episodes if you can see them coming. Again, speak with your child's psychiatrist.

~

If your child has meltdowns or sensory issues when in a particular place (a specific playground or room), avoid that location for a period of two weeks, and then reintroduce it. This will provide a clue as to what is causing the trouble. For example, a particular playground might be too noisy or crowded for him to handle at this time. This happened to Alex. He had a terrible meltdown one day in a park near our apartment. Every time he went near it he would relive the event and tantrum. I kept him away for a period of more than two weeks, and then began to walk near the park. After several trips near the park we finally entered and began to be able to utilize the park again. I have come across this type of "reliving" experience many times and it makes sense. You tie a place, sound, or taste to a pleasing or not pleasing experience. If this happens, work over time to distance from the memory then reintroduce.

This fits along with becoming an expert on your child. You must figure out what triggers a "bad" or disruptive behavior and what elicits a positive behavior. So, what does your child find stressful? Calming? Uncomfortable? Enjoyable? If you understand what affects your child, you'll be better at troubleshooting problems and preventing situations that cause difficulties.

~

Observe your son's behavior and mood following meals, environment changes (going outside during the summer), and exposure to different lighting, sounds, and sights. Become Sherlock Holmes to pinpoint situations that need adjusting.

~

Keep a calm home environment and a good family atmosphere. An overstressed home will not allow a child with autism—who may have ADD, ADHD, and/or sensory processing issues—the secure and tranquil atmosphere he needs. Parents should try to create a harmonious and democratic family atmosphere. If the parents don't get along very well, the child will feel the tension.

~

Don't be afraid to discipline your child when necessary. It is important not to underestimate your child. Children with autism are capable of willful misbehavior. It can be a challenge to determine what is willful and what is not, but parents should not assume that all behaviors are unintentional. Much like a typical child, an autistic child can and should be told what he should or should not do.

~

Becoming Sensory Savvy

Sensory issues can often be mistaken for behavioral problems. Most, if not all kids on the spectrum have some sensory challenges and often recognizing and addressing them will alleviate many behavioral issues. Below are some tips to help you become sensory savvy. Do consult with your child's OT on creating a sensory diet though. While a massage may be calming, given at the wrong time in the wrong place for too long a time, it can be counterproductive and actually increase sensitivity. So don't just try and figure out on your own!

~

If a child has vestibular and visual issues, which impact his perception of his position in space, he might have great difficulty sitting upright in a chair without falling from time to time. To avoid falls or embarrassment, he might fidget to better process his body, or get out of his seat often. He, in turn, will present as a child who "won't" stay seated.

—*Markus Jarrow, "Occupational Therapy and Sensory Integration,"* Cutting-Edge Therapies for Autism

~

With children with sensory integration dysfunction, it is important to remember that these behaviors might be nothing more than effective coping mechanisms. When the underlying sensory issues are addressed, the behavior might disappear altogether.

> —*Markus Jarrow, "Occupational Therapy and Sensory Integration,"* Cutting-Edge Therapies for Autism

~

Children inherently attempt to provide themselves with what they need and avoid what they are frightened by. They constantly listen to their bodies and try to regulate themselves. By listening to what their bodies tell us, we can help them to make a great deal of positive change.

> —*Markus Jarrow, "Occupational Therapy and Sensory Integration,"* Cutting-Edge Therapies for Autism

~

Something you can do to improve eye contact is to be consistent in asking your son to look at your face whenever he wants something. You may not get it every time, but keep to it and respond quicker when he gives you eye contact. He will notice this and work to improve.

More on eye contact: When he asks for an object, hold it directly in front of your face and request eye contact. When he looks to retrieve the object, use affect to reward his glance and make a game of it. Again, consistency is key; keep to it and he will make progress.

~

Make use of self-stimulating behaviors. While stimming is typically performed to gain a sensory escape or satisfy a physical need, if you join in during these periods you may gain a quick glance or other feedback and have the beginning of a communication base to build on.

~

If your son is hyperactive and out of control, don't be tempted to react by shouting to get him to stop; in an overcrowded or noisy location (playground, store), it is likely that the environment is overstimulating him to begin with, and shouting will only make things worse. Likewise, a sensation-craving kid might grab items off a store shelf or run around because the environment is so tempting and overwhelming to his regulatory ability. Scolding will only add to the turmoil and lead to feelings of guilt (by both) later on. To calm the child and get him regulated, remove him from the location, and use a soothing activity such as ice, a swing, music, or deep pressure to aid in calming. Once calm, discuss what happened and why, with understanding. If your child is nonverbal, be more intuitive; use pictures, images, or communication devices to discuss it. Provide him with solutions going forward, or the ability to request pressure or removal from an affecting environment. Always remember to counterbalance a child's loss of control with calm words and gestures, and help the child reorganize and regain focus and attention.

—Stanley Greenspan, MD, *Overcoming ADHD*

Alternatively, the child might need you to be completely quiet.

~

So, listen to your child's body language: Is he running, jumping, crashing onto the floor or into the wall? Does he prefer sedentary activities? Talk to your child's occupational therapist about the movements and sensations that your child seeks. Ask for a sensory diet to give your child consistent input and help satisfy these "cravings."

~

Put your child to work. Heavy work that includes resistive activities (such as pushing, pulling, and carrying) provides input that is organizing and calming. At home you can have your child help with everyday chores while providing this important information to the body. Examples: pushing in chairs after mealtimes, pushing shopping carts at the grocery store, carrying heavier food items (rice, cans, etc.) and helping to put them away, carrying boxes of games to clean up, pulling the laundry basket to the machine, etc.

~

We use our mouths to help us stay regulated and calm (think gum, sucking candies, biting your lip, or chewing the inside of your cheek). Give your child oral input by using straws to drink thick shakes, yogurt, applesauce, pudding, etc. Cut straws shorter if it is too difficult. Use narrower or longer straws to increase the challenge. Provide chewy (e.g., dried fruit) and crunchy foods (e.g., apples). This facilitates oral motor development while providing heavy work for the mouth. Talk to your child's speech or occupational therapist about other ways to provide oral input.

Clothing Sensory Issues

Below are some tips on avoiding sensory troubles that can be associated with clothing.

- Consider using 100 percent cotton clothing.
- Wash clothing and bedding with non-allergenic soaps (no dyes, no additives).
- What do you do with a child who strips off his clothes at every opportunity? First, you try to find out why. The most common reason is sensory sensitivity, so first talk to an occupational therapist about instituting a program of sensory integration therapy.
- In the meantime, see what you can do to make staying clothed more comfortable. Verbal children may be able to explain what they don't like about wearing clothes.

Common problems include chafing waistbands, itchy fabrics, "new-clothes" smell, and annoying tags. Kids who can't stand regular waistbands can often handle elastic-waist pants and shorts, especially those made with soft fabrics, such as sweatpants. Others can wear only overalls or coveralls with ease, and these have the added "bonus" of being harder to remove.

- For children who wear diapers, the diaper itself may be the problem. Check for and treat any actual diaper rash. (Incidentally, diaper rash can be caused by a yeast infection on the skin, which may indicate a larger problem with yeast overgrowth.) Experiment with different types of cloth diapers, various brands of disposables, and larger diapers if tightness around the waist and legs is an issue.

- Explore catalogs that carry special clothing for children with disabilities. Many items in these catalogs are especially good for older children who have toileting problems, or for children with orthopedic impairments in addition to an ASD.

- Many people with sensory problems prefer soft fabrics, such as cotton jersey or terrycloth, over stiff fabrics like denim. If this is the case with your child, go shopping with that in mind. It can help to wash new clothing a few times before wearing it, to remove that stiff feeling as well as any unfamiliar smells.

- If an aversion to clothing crops up suddenly, make sure you haven't just changed your detergent or fabric softener. There may be a smell or allergy issue going on.

- Remove tags from inside of garments as needed.

- One solution that will save you money and hassles is purchasing used clothing instead of new ones. These pre-softened garments may already feel "just right." Again, they may need to be washed a few times to take away any bothersome scents.

Showing Affection to Your Child with Sensory-Processing Issues

Never underestimate the power of a hug. Bear hugs show affection while giving your child input that helps them learn about their bodies to build better body awareness. This input is grounding and calming. Remember, light touch tends to be aversive, so when giving hugs, placing your hand on a shoulder, or rubbing your child's back, deep, firm pressure is the way to go, as long as it is safe. Don't be surprised if your child starts asking for more "hugs," "squeezes," and "rubs." If he resists hugs, talk to an OT about other ways to provide this input. Here are some tips from Cathy Purple Cherry on more ways to show affection.

Tips by Cathy Purple Cherry, AIA, LEED AP

- Affection can be shown to all people through words and imagery, not just through touch. Thus, surround your sensitive child with words and images of love.

- Understand the sensory issues of your ASD child to avoid using or wearing materials that trigger a negative response. This may allow you to have successful physical contact.

- Try approaching your child from various levels— maybe not standing full height but on your knees. You may find the point of initial touch changes the ASD child's response. You can even try lying down with your child before touching him. Also try various body areas for successful touch using different kinds of pressure. It may be that simple pressure to the top of the head where hair provides a layer of insulation is the best touch.

- It may be difficult to accept that you cannot snuggle up to your autistic son or that he does not appear to be bonding with you. Work on accepting this fact yourself so that you do not go through your child's life feeling rejected. He did not ask to be born with these challenges.

- When physical affection isn't an option, try the following: use music and dance to show love as long as auditory processing sensitivities do not exist.

- Give something yummy to eat to show that you love him, and decorate it regardless of what it is. Remember the small things that reminded you your mother loved you. A peanut butter and jelly sandwich cut with heart-shaped cookie cutters is a good thing.

- As you work to build levels of affection with your ASD child and get comfortable with the strategies above (or any that you create on your own) that work, do not neglect to inform caregivers and other family members about what you are doing. One weekend with the grandparents who may not be on the same page could cause a regression and undermine all your hard work.

Holiday Season

The following tips are adapted from "Twelve Tips for Helping People with Autism and Their Families Have a Happy Holiday" by the Autism Society of America, www.autism-society.org/holiday_tips.

Preparation is crucial for many individuals. At the same time, it is important to determine how much preparation a specific person may need. For example, if your son has a tendency to become anxious when anticipating an event that is to occur in the future, you may want to adjust how many days in advance you prepare him. Preparation can occur in various ways, by using a calendar and marking the dates of various holiday events, or by creating a social story that highlights what will happen at a given event.

~

Decorations around the house may be disruptive for some. It may be helpful to revisit pictures from previous holidays that show decorations in the house. If such a photo book does not exist, use this holiday season to create one. For some it may also be helpful to take them shopping with you for holiday decorations so that they are engaged in the process, or involve them in the process of decorating the house. And once holiday decorations have been put up, you may need to create rules about those that can and cannot be touched. Be direct, specific, and consistent.

If a person with autism has difficulty with change, you may want to gradually decorate the house. For example, on the first day, put up the Christmas tree; then on the next day, decorate the tree; and so on. And again, engage them as much as possible in this process. It may be helpful to develop a visual schedule or calendar that shows what will be done on each day.

~

If a person with autism begins to obsess about a particular gift or item they want, it may be helpful to be specific and direct about the number of times they can mention the gift. One suggestion is to give them five chips. They are allowed to exchange one chip for five minutes of talking about the desired gift. Also, if you have no intention of purchasing a specific item, it serves no purpose to tell them that maybe they will get the gift. This will only lead to problems in the future. Always choose to be direct and specific about your intentions.

Practice opening gifts, taking turns and waiting for others, and giving gifts. Role-play scenarios with your child in preparation for him getting a gift he does not want. Talk through this process to avoid embarrassing moments with family members. You might also choose to practice certain religious rituals. Work with a speech-language pathologist to construct pages of vocabulary or topic boards that relate to the holidays and family traditions.

~

Teach them how to leave a situation and/or how to access support when an event becomes overwhelming. For example, if you are having visitors, have a space set aside for the child as his safe/calm space. The individual should be taught ahead of time that they should go to their space when feeling overwhelmed. This self-management tool will serve the individual into adulthood. For those who are not at that level of self-management, develop a signal or cue for them to show when they are getting anxious, and prompt them to use the space. For individuals with more significant challenges, practice using this space in a calm manner at various times prior to your guests' arrival. Take them into the room and engage them in calming activities (e.g., play soft music, rub his back, turn down the lights, etc.). Then when you notice the individual becoming anxious, calmly remove him from the anxiety provoking setting immediately and take him into the calming environment.

~

If you are traveling for the holidays, make sure you have your son's favorite foods or items available. Having familiar items readily available can help to calm stressful situations. Also, prepare him via social stories or other communication systems for any unexpected delays in travel. If you are flying for the first time, it may be helpful to bring him to the airport in advance and help him to become accustomed to airports and planes. Use social stories and pictures to rehearse what will happen when boarding and flying.

~

Prepare a photo album of the relatives and other guests who will be visiting during the holidays in advance. Allow the person with autism access to these photos at all times and also go through the photo album with him while talking briefly about each family member.

Prepare family members for strategies to use to minimize anxiety or behavioral incidents, and to enhance participation. Help them to understand if the person with autism needs calm discussions, and if he prefers to be hugged/kissed or not. Provide other suggestions that will facilitate a smoother holiday season.

~

If the person with autism is on special diet, make sure there is food available that he can eat. And even if he is not on a special diet, be cautious of the amount of sugar consumed. And try to maintain a sleep and meal routine.

~

Above all, know your loved one with autism. Know how much noise and other sensory input he can take. Know his level of anxiety and the amount of preparation it may take. Know his fears and those things that will make the season more enjoyable for him. Don't stress. Plan in advance. And most of all, have a wonderful holiday season!

Before a Holiday Event

- Create a social story or draw pictures of what the holiday is about and what the party/dinner will be like. In particular, the number of people involved, and sensory impact of decorations, music, lighting, etc.

- Practice sitting at the table with all objects (plates, utensils) and ambiance (music, lighting) in place.
- Modify as many foods as possible to accommodate diets. Remember the diets for ASD kids are not like those of a fitness or weight loss regime, where occasional cheats are possible. Diets such as the SCD diet are more akin to peanut allergies. In many cases the foods restricted make our kids sick, and are not something to cheat on.
- If the environment is not ASD friendly, create an area your child can retreat to. For instance, allocate a bedroom for him and turn down the lighting, perhaps put on calming music, and maybe even his own snacks. Perhaps include blankets and other helpful items to combat the potential stress in other areas of the home. Have guests 'visit' your son there, one at a time, to help integrate him into the event.
- Likewise, have alternative activities for the ASD child if he is averse to what the overall holiday activity might be (e.g., watching the game on TV at Thanksgiving).
- Practice event behaviors in advance such as getting kissed, shaking hands, lighting or blowing out candles, opening gifts, etc.
- If the child is anxious about gifts, keep all hidden till the last moment before opening.

- Keep a calendar or countdown till the day of the event, such as the tree is coming in six days, or five days till we open presents.
- Get some sensory suggestions from your son's OT and other therapists about handling holidays.

More Tips for surviving the holidays:

The winter holidays and celebrations can be difficult for children on the spectrum and their families. Some areas of difficulty include:

- The stores are full of noise, lights, lots of people, and winter holiday music that can create major overwhelm for those with sensory processing challenges.
- Social requirements such as visiting relatives wanting a hug or a kiss that can feel painful.
- Holiday dinners where he is expected to try foods or sit for long periods of time with so many people and so much commotion.
- Many children are mesmerized by the colors and textures of the ribbon and wrapping paper and do not open the present but stim on (get engrossed in playing with) the wrapping.
- The child does not understand personal space or have notions of safety and so he may run around the house or handle something breakable.

- Relatives may think the that the child is misbehaving, and may try to discipline the child, not realizing that the child really can't help it, and that discipline is not helpful when it comes to sensory overload and high anxiety.

- Parents have a difficult time because they know there are certain expectations of behavior that relatives and friends have and that the child cannot fulfill.

~

What can you do? Here are some tips on how to prepare your friends and relatives whom you will be visiting:

- Explain the difficulties your child has with the holiday dinner environment, decorations, noise, etc.

- Let your friends and relatives know that he is not just misbehaving, and that he is learning little by little how to handle these situations.

- Explain about dietary challenges so they don't expect him to eat what everyone else is eating.

- Ask if there is a quiet room (child-proof in terms of décor) where your child can retreat for some quiet time to escape the commotion and noise.

- Send them a short but sweet letter or email explaining why your child acts the way he does and the difficulties of the holidays from his point of view. They will have a better understanding of why he won't wear a necktie, and why as more and more people start arriving, he tries to escape the room.

~

To prepare your child ahead of time:

- Make a social stories book about what will be happening and the behavioral expectations. If possible include photos of who he will be seeing and the house as it was decorated at last year's holiday season. If he is going to church, do the same for that environment.
- Play some of the music he may be hearing at this holiday season.
- Practice unwrapping presents—wrap a bunch of boxes up with his favorite treats inside and have him open them to get to them.
- Practice a handshake if he can tolerate that.
- Write rules together—i.e., how long he thinks he can tolerate sitting at table, and expected behavior.

~

On the day of the holiday celebration:

- Remind your child of the agreed upon rules.
- Pack some little toys he can play with in his lap at the dinner table.
- Bring some foods he can eat, especially if he is on a specific diet.

- Arrive early so that the noise level builds up slowly for him.

- Do not let the expectations of others ruin your day. Do what you need to do to make it as comfortable as possible for you and your child.

—Chantal Sicile-Kira (www.chantalsicile-kira.com)

Toys & Gifts

Often, simple, everyday items present successfully as toys. Empty boxes and a roll of tape are simple and safe and work great to provide hours of activity. Dangling keys making interesting noises can be intriguing to some ASD children though others will try and place them in any holes and cause possible damage. Old wallets provide hidden compartments for folded paper and collected treasures found from the ground. One of my son's favorite things is duct tape as he makes numerous objects or transforms old things into new play shapes. The behavior of repeating actions was very satisfying to him. Thus taping and re-taping and re-taping provided him with hours of interest.

~

Though this may already be obvious, textured toys can provide great tactile stimulation and squishy toys can provide stress reduction. But, if you don't want the liquid of a squishy toy all over your house, don't give them one filled with liquid. They WILL figure out a way to get it out. The same goes for the textured toys. Picking may be something your child likes to do so do not provide a tactile toy with a well-raised texture as these elements will be picked off.

Chewy toys can take care of that oral fixation, but are also quite durable. They are easy to carry wherever you go. Check out SensoryUniversity.com. Also, ask your OT for suggestions.

~

Sorting things is, at times, very appealing to autistic children as it allows them to organize their world. Thus, depending upon the age of the child, the toys for this application could be very different. For the younger children, colored blocks would work. For the older child, it may be buttons or coins.

~

Some things to keep in mind:

- Little parts on toys are not a good thing. They can cause frustration and, more significantly, stimulate the interest to take the toy apart.
- Loud, noisy toys do not work—not just because of their possible annoyance to your ASD child but because they may stimulate activity and behaviors that you are trying to reduce.

- Do not provide toys with any sharp corners or edges at any age because, during tantrums, these objects can become weapons both to the autistic child and towards their siblings or your home.

Dining Out Tips

Avoid long—or, let's face it, any—restaurant waits. Go early or late to avoid any crowds. The last thing you want is a pre-meal meltdown. Try diners; we have found them to be accommodating, and they have a wide range of options.

Anyplace that has an outside seating option is great; less hassle with cleanup, should your son be a messy eater like Alex, and you can always take a walk.

~

Make sure the restaurant can accommodate whatever diet your child is on. This is not always easy. Google the menu and then call to confirm ingredients and how the meal you'll be ordering is prepared. Mention allergies, and make clear that MSG is off limits.

Once you find a good place that's suitable for your child, become a regular and tip well. In the future you'll be able to call and make special requests, or even order in advance.

~

You can ease your way into eating out. First, I took Alex to some out-of-the-way places just to get french fries. Then, I took him to restaurants at less-popular times and ordered full meals. Finally, we worked toward having a regular meal out at dinnertime.

This takes time. To get him to a comfortable place dining out, I worked on this routine for about four months, leading up to his birthday. On the big day he was able to remain regulated, and I was able to actually enjoy eating out. Practice makes perfect.

You can also prepare for eating out by watching Elmo or other favorite characters eat out on TV or YouTube, and discussing how you will both be doing the same.

~

Once you are seated and you've ordered, pay your bill ahead of time. Give the waiter your card and mention the possibility of having to leave early.

As with travel, bring some items to help with any waits. YouTube on an iPhone works for us, but books and chewy toys can also serve the purpose.

Feel free to mention autism at the start of the meal to anyone working your table; it will help the staff understand, and you'll be able to relax.

Vacations and Travel Tips

Remember to plan your vacations around your child's interests. Alex loves the water and being outdoors, so I focus on places with a pool and access to hiking trails. You can usually plan many nice day trips to national parks or scenic local areas.

Vacation in a national park. Think about it: You bring your own food, so no worry about diet violations; it's cost-effective, beautiful, and a wonderful way to connect with your son and to nature. There is something soothing and stabilizing about hiking in the great outdoors. There are many fabulous parks located throughout the United States. Check out www.nps.gov/findapark/index. htm.

"In every walk with nature one receives far more than he seeks."

—John Muir

~

Some cruise lines now have cruises specially designated for children with autism and their families. Just Google "autism cruises."

~

Plenty of rest time at the hotel is one of the keys to a successful vacation. And putting a cap on the number of activities per day should help to prevent meltdowns.

~

Ask your OT for an "on-the-go" sensory box to help your child proactively remain regulated on flights or long car trips. A shoebox or Ziploc with Play-Doh, squish balls, etc., definitely comes in handy.

~

Off-peak weeks at theme parks mean shorter lines, smaller crows, and less noise. Plan accordingly. And don't forget to bring earplugs or headphones for your kid for when the loud noises get to be too much for him.

~

Asking a doctor, therapist, or teacher for a letter addressed to the airline that states the child's diagnosis and challenges can cut down on wait time getting on and off a flight. Being able to hand a typed letter to someone rather than talking about your child in front of them is always a better option, especially during difficult times in the air.

Traveling is all about Transitions

Preparing the person—child, teenager, or adult—as much as possible will make any trip a more enjoyable experience for all involved. Some advance planning of specific steps of the trip can be made ahead of time to prepare both the person and the environment for a better travel experience.

> *Here are some tips from Chantal Sicile-Kira, www. chantalsicile-kira.com for that better experience.*
>
> - Think of the individual's daily routine and the items he likes or needs and bring them along to make him feel more at home. Bring whatever foods and drinks will keep him happy on the trip, especially if there are dietary restrictions.
> - Buy some small, inexpensive toys or books that he can play with during the journey (and if you lose them, it won't be the end of the world). If he only plays with one favorite item, try to find a duplicate and see if you can "break it in" before the trip.
> - Do not wash any items (including plush toys) before the trip, as the individual may feel comfort in the "home" smell of his cherished item.
> - Put up a monthly calendar with the departure date clearly marked, and have the person check off every day until departure. Bring the calendar with you and mark off the number of days in one place or on the trip, always having the return date indicated.

- Put together a picture and word "travel book" of what means of transport you are going to be using, who you are going to see, where you will sleep, and what you will do or see at your destination(s). Go over this with the person, like you would a storybook, as often as you like in preparation for the trip. Using a three-ring binder is best, as you can add extra pages or insert the calendar mentioned above for use on the trip.

- Put together a picture or word schedule of the actual journey to take with you on your trip. Add extra pages to the travel book. Add Velcro and attach pictures or words in order of the travel sequence. For example, a picture to represent the car ride to the airport, going through security, getting on the airplane, etc. For car trips, pictures representing different stops on the trip and number of miles to be driven can be used. Add an empty envelope to add the "done" pictures when you have finished one step of the journey.

- Taking a short trip before attempting longer ones is recommended, if possible. This will help the person get used to traveling and give you the opportunity to plan ahead for possible areas of difficulty. Also, if you use the travel book system, it will help the person make a connection between the travel book and any impending travel in the future.

- When staying in a hotel, it is a good idea to call ahead and ask for a quiet room. You may wish to explain about the person's behavior if there is a likelihood of him or her exhibiting such behavior in the public part of the hotel. Same with a friend or relative's home; it can be a bit disconcerting for everyone concerned if your child or adolescent takes his clothes off and races through your friend's home stark naked.

- If you are traveling by plane, call the airline, as far in advance as you can, and tell them you will be traveling with someone who has special needs. Some airlines have "special assistance coordinators." You may wish to explain about the person's needs and some of the behaviors that may affect other travelers, such as rocking in their seat. If the person is a rocker, asking for bulkhead seats or the last row of seats on the plane will limit the number of fellow travelers that are impacted by the rocking. If you need assistance getting the person and luggage to the gate, or to change planes during the trip, call ahead and reserve wheelchair assistance. Even if the person does not need a wheelchair, this guarantees that someone will be waiting for you and available to assist you.

- Persons with autism should always carry identification. Make sure he has an ID tag attached to him somewhere, with a current phone number written on it. You can order medical bracelets, necklaces, and tags to attach to shoelaces. Additionally, if the person can carry it in his pocket, make an ID card with a current photo, date, and phone numbers. Be sure to include any other important information, such as allergies and medications, and any special information (i.e., nonverbal).

- Adult passengers (eighteen and over) are required to show a US federal or state-issued photo ID that contains the following information: name, date of birth, gender, expiration date, and a tamper-resistant feature in order to be allowed to go through the checkpoint and onto their flight. Acceptable identification includes: driver's license or other state photo identity card issued by the Department of Motor Vehicles (or equivalent) that meets REAL ID benchmarks (at time of writing, all states are currently in compliance).

Living with Your Autistic Child in Your Home

Tips by Cathy Purple Cherry, AIA, LEED AP

When an autistic child has siblings, especially younger ones, there can be considerable conflict that occurs in a home environment. There are simple practical design solutions and strategies that can be applied to your home to help reduce this conflict.

If you are designing a home from scratch, aside from implementing ADA strategies such as wider door openings, ramps, and ADA-approved light and plumbing fixtures for possible physical challenges your child may have, the following design items should be considered for the autism spectrum:

- Increase the floor area between the kitchen counter and the kitchen island to a minimum of five to six feet. This helps improve the personal space of the family members and reduce the potential for touching and a sense of invasion.

- If the house is a larger scale, include two staircases with each staircase a minimum of four feet in width to help reduce the possibility of path crossing.

- Provide an en suite bathroom to the autistic child's bedroom. This eliminates the gross-out factor that can happen between two siblings, which is further amplified by the inappropriate judgment of the ASD child and the inappropriate reactions of the sibling.

- Install an electric oven. Do not install gas. Curiosity with fire can be an issue with ASD children and teens, and this helps eliminate the risk of feeding that curiosity.

- Use wood flooring, not carpet, so that you can hear the footsteps of the child or teen and understand their movements in your home. This gives you as a parent a chance to prevent conflict and poor judgment.

- Install wood blocking behind drywall for all towel and robe hooks. The toggle bolts do not hold up to the strength of these individuals and their misjudgment in removing items from these hooks as they get older.

- Install plywood behind the drywall and hallway areas or in their room to help prevent damage to the walls as oppositional behaviors develop during adolescence.

- Overall, remember impulsivity leads to inappropriate decisions and conflict. The best strategy is "out of sight, out of mind." I learned this after our ASD son pulled a knife from a knife block visible on the kitchen counter and used it as a weapon to threaten someone at the age of ten. If you do not want my son to touch, steal, impulsively take or break something, then you must keep things out of sight. Keep all knives in a cabinet, all lighters hidden, all tools in a closet or in a secured area, all firearms and firecrackers in safes, and all money locked away.

~

If your home already exists, the following ideas can still be implemented:

Create a separate snack cabinet in the kitchen to prevent the siblings from being grossed out by the touching of shared food. When siblings are young, they have not yet developed the ability to respond appropriately to their autistic sibling. As is true in our home, this situation is compounded when the siblings are younger than the ASD teen.

~

Clearly define the outdoor play area for the ASD child. This area can be demarcated by plantings, structures, or sculptures. Defining this area allows the individual with special needs to do anything they desire without conflict with the other siblings also playing in the same yard.

~

Provide a preset number of drawers in the child's room for hoarded objects. Explain that if the drawers get filled, the child must remove objects to make more room for other items.

~

Completely eliminate the door locks specifically on the ASD child's bathroom, as well as bedroom. Our son likes to lock himself in the bathroom when he is having a fit. He is also known to stand outside his shower and pretend to bathe by wetting his hair. Without the lock, this allows me to knock on the door and then enter and check to see what he is doing.

~

Place timers in the ASD child's bedroom, bathroom, and the kitchen. Using timers aids in giving the individual a better sense of how long something should take. Matthew has no sense of time whatsoever. We started using these in his bathroom, as his showers were forty minutes long. These timers aided in Matthew learning better judgment as to how long something should take. We no longer use them, but do still at times need to prompt him or count down.

~

Place locks on certain cabinets to help control access to items that present dangers. Further, there may be obsessions with specific food items that need to be managed by placing these foods in these cabinets.

~

If necessary, set up the autistic teen's room like a college dormitory, providing relative independence from the rest of the house. As our son has gotten older, his strength has increased but his judgment has not improved. For the safety of our other children who are younger and smaller, it is necessary to strategize how to reduce the overlapping paths of our kids. We have discussed this strategy, as mealtime is definitely one of the worst times in our home due to the table manners, voice tone, poor reactions, and inappropriate behaviors of our ASD son.

Productive Approaches to Parenting

Having autism does not mean your son cannot have a fulfilling life; do not allow the language of victimhood into your vocabulary. Use empowering words that teach him that he is without limits. Here are some tips to help with getting though the day and educating at the same time.

~

Work to give your child some structured chores he can work on each day. This will help increase the structure in his day and give him a feeling of accomplishment each day. We suggest placing play items in a home bin and helping with laundry.

Now these chores may not be easy to define or organize at first, but stick to it, let him have some responsibility and build on it. You may feel compelled to do the task yourself, but give him time to get the hang of it and you'll both be rewarded. As with any facet of autism, you will need a little patience.

Giving intermediate goalposts creates more opportunities for engagement and feelings of accomplishment.

A clearly defined daily schedule for your son can work wonders to remove uncertainty and accompanying frustration, for you both!

~

If you are completely honest with yourself about your child's strengths and weaknesses, you can more effectively advocate on his behalf. Self-delusion is a luxury you can't afford.

~

Don't get caught in the heat of the moment. When speaking, always take a breath and deliver a measured response.

~

Be flexible regarding timing. If your child moves away from brushing his hair, rather than forcing or pushing it, wait ten minutes and try again.

Flexibility is key, especially when it comes to timing. Knowing when to back off and when to return to a task or duty is more art than science. Keeping a flexible mindset and being persistent will help!

~

Try not to become overprotective. This is easy to do and easier to understand, but it is counterproductive. If you give your son control of a situation or at least expand his control of a situation, you can give him a "wow" moment where he can adapt and learn.

~

Keep yourself in a happy place. Easier said than done many times, I know. But your emotions have significant repercussions on your son, which should serve as a reminder and motive to keep things as positive as possible. Eliminate all negative influences, thoughts, and people if necessary. You and your son don't have time for negativity!

Seek some good self time and solace. Go for a walk in the woods, run in the park, or read a book by a lake. You need to take care of yourself and activities in nature have a tonic effect.

Building Self-Esteem

Remember, as much as possible, treat your children as though they were typically developing. Kids will always live up to your lowest expectations. Here are some tips to help.

~

Raise your son to have good self-esteem, a necessary trait for a successful life. This means raising him with the firm knowledge that you love him and believe in him. Set high expectations for your boy, but give him the means to reach them. Teach him that he has the right to his own opinion, and respect the choices he makes when he is given the opportunity to choose. Raise him to believe that with hard work, he can reach his goals. In this way, he can reach his true potential.

—*Chantal Sicile-Kira, author of* Autism Life Skills,
www.chantalsicile-kira.com

~

Children develop most of their self-esteem based on what they hear and experience at home. Take a day and listen to the "messages" your boy is hearing at home. Does he hear mostly positive remarks or negative remarks? Is he accepted for who he is while still being expected to reach his potential? Is he complimented for all the positive things he does (and not just criticized for the negative behaviors)? Words and attitude do make a difference.

~

Parents should not allow autism to define their child. Just as one would not narrowly define a child with high blood sugar by saying "My child is diabetes," a child with autistic features and manifestations should not be labeled "autism." Your child is not autism. Your child is a sweet and wonderful individual who, just like all of us, has multiple positive attributes and a variety of challenges that need to be addressed.

—Dr. Mark Freilich, Total Kids Developmental
Pediatric Resources, New York City

Organization

This is a key task. The days of parents of autistic kids are hectic enough; we don't need to be looking for items throughout the day. Work to develop an organized mindset. Often we are too tired by the end of day to do any heavy thinking or mental work. So that time is ideal for organization tasks: putting things in their place, marking off checklists, to do lists, and filling out that spreadsheet I keep talking about. Here are some more tips to help get organized.

∼

Creating a bin system for your child's supplies and toys can be useful. Separate the types of toys and supplies into individual bins, then take photographs of each type of toy or supply contained within and tape the photograph to the front of each corresponding bin.

∼

Openly display children's toys, supplies, and clothing. It is easier for autistic children to stay organized and function if they can see all of their belongings. Drawers do not usually work well for children on the autism spectrum. Hang as many of their clothes as possible, or fold them and place them on shelves, preferably cubbies. Place jeans in one cubby, sweatshirts in another, and so on. Socks, underwear, and pajamas are best placed in transparent bins with photographs taped to the front. If you don't have cubbies, you may tape photographs on the front of each drawer. If possible, do not combine items into one drawer.

~

Set up daily routines and stick to them as much as possible. Creating regular daily routines can make transitioning from one activity to another less upsetting. Children on the autism spectrum often thrive when they have daily routines and usually react poorly to changes in routines. Once a solid routine is created, small changes can be introduced slowly, and can help your child develop coping strategies to deal with transitions. Note: it is best to introduce changes in routines in very small steps. Gradually, your child will be able to use strategies like social stories and self-talk to work through the anxiety they experience when making transitions.

An example of an organizing routine is to give your child a ten-minute heads-up before dinner each evening, and then have them set a timer for ten minutes. Teach them that when the timer goes off, they are to pick up all of their toys and place them in the appropriate bins. This establishes a routine, lets them know what to expect, gives them a ten-minute lead time, and then provides them with a distinct audio clue when it's time to pick up and get organized.

An addition to this routine could be that when the timer goes off and it's time to pick up and get organized, you could play a specific song that your child would come to recognize as the "pick up and get organized" song. This can make it fun, playful, and soothing, and can also help keep them on task so they will get the work done faster.

Finally, create a visual schedule for your child. Picture schedules work best for autistic kids. Set up the picture schedule so that when your child is finished with the task/activity, they can move that picture to the "all-done" side. Essentially, you are creating an interactive picture schedule that your child can "control." Their picture schedule could also be organized by first, next, last. It will give them the order of tasks, and, once completed, they can move the picture to the "completed" side. There are many apps that can help with this.

Managing a Treatment Team

From a management perspective, it is most efficient to have one parent "in charge of autism." Many times one parent will be more focused on the effort and thus have more information at hand. That individual should make the calls, while providing full disclosure to the other. The other parent should focus on other children in the family, or, in the case of a single child, a specific task—say, biomedical research, or planning family outings.

~

As you move forward in your treatments, school selection, and other endeavors, do not become wedded to any one institution or individual. Things will change with your child over time and you will need to monitor and adjust programs and individuals accordingly. Be flexible and constantly seek improvements.

~

Remember to develop relationships with the teachers, doctors, and therapists who work with your son. Share information often; consider yourself the "team" leader. I think of myself as CEO of team Alex and regularly have communications with all those who work with Alex. I also put various members of the team in touch with each other and try to have periodic meetings. A good idea is to have a "party" and invite the team over to have some fun and go over progress, areas for improvement, and getting all members on the same page.

Communicate with all of the individuals who are part of the team educating your child. By developing a team atmosphere or approach and consistently using structured programs, your son will receive the best treatment possible. All individuals involved in this team structure need to work together to reach common goals.

Every member of the team needs to agree on the program, goals and treatment for the child. Open communication is also essential. This ensures that everyone is working together to achieve the same objectives, which provides consistency and reinforcement of the objectives.

~

Document everything. Scan and make copies of printed forms and print any online forms in case you need them during phone calls and meetings. You will continually call upon all of your autism documents, notes, and records. Organizing your documents will also improve communication between a multidisciplinary health team— not to mention reduce your stress levels.

~

A treatment program containing a greater number of therapies or therapists does not necessarily mean better treatment. Having a smaller number of treatment providers can allow for deeper relationships between child and therapists, and parents and therapists. The more therapists who work with your boy with ASD, the more likely [your child will be] fragmented.

—Lauren Tobing-Puente, PhD, Licensed Psychologist,
www.drtobingpuente.com

~

Your child should always be happy to see his/her therapist. If not, reevaluate the therapy *and* provider. Often times the therapy is not the issue, but who is performing it.

Trust your gut when seeking a new treatment provider. You should feel comfortable very early on with your son's therapists. Even those with the best reputations do not always mean the best fit for your son, you, and your family.

—Lauren Tobing-Puente, PhD, Licensed Psychologist,
www.drtobingpuente.com

One measure of a therapist's effectiveness is your child's progress. Is your child experiencing success with this therapist? If not, why? Watch the way your child reacts to the therapist during a treatment session, and vice versa. Is your child happy [to be with the therapist]? Is the therapist happy [to be with your child]?

—Karen Siff Exkorn, The Autism Sourcebook

Toilet Training

Another issue for many kids on the spectrum, and this one tends to cause parents much frustration and lost sleep. My son was not fully trained till he was eleven years old. It was a long battle to figure out causality and find the right strategies, but we did it! Below are some tips that were helpful to others and us.

~

If you are having problems with nighttime wettings, you may need to increase the frequency of bathroom visits. Set your alarm for every hour or two and bring him to the bathroom even if he appears to not have to go. As you get drier nights, extend the time between visits until you are all good for the evening. Do not get discouraged by the occasional backslide. My son had this problem for years and in about a month I was able to transition him to no pull-ups and sleeping through the night.

~

FYI: Some meds, most notably risperidone/Risperdal, have the side effect of lessening urination control. Check your meds and review side effects.

~

Targeting—you can use a target or just try an ice cube. While ice works well, if you Google "toilet targets," or search on Amazon you will find several actual products that can be placed in the bowl to provide a visual target and potentially be fun for your son.

~

A common problem is that a child might be able to use the toilet correctly at home but refuse to use it at school. This might be due to a failure to recognize the toilet. Hilde De Clercq from Belgium discovered that an autistic child might use a small nonrelevant detail to recognize an object such as a toilet. It takes detective work to find that detail. In one case a boy would only use the toilet at home that had a black seat. His parents and teacher were able to get him to use the toilet at school by covering its white seat with black tape. The tape was then gradually removed and toilets with white seats became recognized as toilets.

—*Temple Grandin, PhD, author of* Thinking in Pictures *and* The Way I See It*; www.autism.com/ind_teaching_tips.asp*

~

If bedwetting remains an issue, rule out allergic bedwetting. If nighttime soiling is a problem, consult a knowledgeable gastroenterologist who has experience with children with autism. This might be a symptom of a gastrointestinal disorder.

~

More Toileting Tips

by Cathy Purple Cherry, AIA, LE

- Children with autism often learn through constantly repeated routines. Thus, the solution to successful toilet training may be tied to repeated practice. Be diligent. When you look back on the many years of rearing an ASD child to adulthood, you will realize "patience" was your child's gift to you! Thus . . . practice and patience, practice and patience, practice and patience x hundreds of times.

- An ASD child is not always aware of his surroundings. Their tactile sensitivities can be somewhat dulled. Our son is minimally affected by heat and cold, for example. Thus recognize that the child may not care if he has made a mess in his clothing. Acceptance by you of this behavior may be the bigger challenge and the only solution.

- A reward system is known to be successful at school for modifying behaviors. Try a point sheet or rewards chart that leads to something good if your child takes steps towards successful toilet training. For our son, during a time in his development, a can of cherry pie filling was more motivating to him than an ice cream sundae, so play to the interests at the time!

- Develop a silent signal between you and your son so that he can quietly communicate his bathroom urges to you before accidents happen. If he uses this signal, reward him.

- Try allowing your autistic child to pee in the grass. This can be fun for all little children and provides the ASD child the practice of not peeing in his pants.

Sleep

Occasional sleep problems can result from many different sources and be difficult to analyze. Look at possible side effects of any new medications, any change in diet, the need for a bowel movement, adjustments to schedule or perhaps too many naps during the day. Once again, a log of daily activities can help pinpoint the cause.

~

Sleep rules! Remember kids and parents perform better and will be happier with a good night's sleep. Do not allow medications or other treatments to limit this important function. Try melatonin if there are difficulties; it works for many kids on the spectrum and suggested for parents having trouble sleeping as well. It also has the benefit of being a potent antitoxin. In addition to melatonin, I've recently discovered hemp (CBD) oil, which has been a real game changer for us in many ways (think no anxiety, for one) but also is beneficial in promoting sleep.

~

Chronic problems can occur in the absence of a consistent bedtime routine, which should include a specific bedtime and a clearly defined sleep location, both a bedroom and a bed. In addition, limit use of TV and devices prior to bed. Alex sleeps well for years now and follows a routine of bath at 8 p.m. (with Epsom salts) followed by melatonin and a ginger based drink. At 9 p.m. devices are off (we do not watch TV) and he is asleep by 9:30 p.m., or 10 p.m. at the latest. We also follow this routine on weekends.

Additionally, you can provide your son with a visual display of bedtime rules, and pair the bedtime rules and routines that you create with reading aloud, which can help address your child's sleep-related anxieties.

~

Regarding those Epsom salt baths. Give in the evening, and morning if time permits. Epsom salt promotes calming and acts as a mild chelator, pulling toxins from the body. It also promotes sleep.

~

Regarding melatonin. Use at night, start with 1 mg, increase the dose as needed and as weight increases. Use the slow-release formulation for night awakenings, standard formulation for trouble falling asleep. This supplement is very safe and easy to go on and off in comparison to sleep drugs. Side benefits include more mellow days (a good night's sleep does wonders) and antioxidant properties.

~

Adjust the home environment for optimal calming. Go green with some plants, notably snake plants, which produce extra oxygen and are easy to care for. In fact, involve your son in their care with adding watering to his chores. Along this line, Himalayan salt crystals, which you can find on Amazon, provide a soft, calming glow and additionally clean the air.

You can also adjust the bedroom environment to make it more appealing to your son. Some kids respond well to having a night-light, while others require total darkness, with a blackout blind over the window to block all exterior light. Many autistic kids sleep better when their bed is pushed up against the wall, as they feel more secure (a corner is even better).

To block out any sounds that may distress your child, use a white-noise machine; run a fan in your child's bedroom; or play Mozart or some other sensory friendly music at a very low volume. Nature sounds, Native American flute music, and chakra chants are very calming and something I highly recommend.

Just remember as you add or try something new, do one thing at a time and keep in consistent for a while, and then add another slowly over time.

~

If you usually sleep in the same bed as your autistic child and he or she is struggling to sleep alone, "replace" yourself with a sleeping bag or body pillow to mimic the pressure that would usually exist if you were lying in the bed.

Additionally, to transition to separate beds you can create a hotel-room setup: trade your king or queen bed for a couple of twins, and put a table in between (after a period of the beds being next to one another) to build sleeping independence. Once they are comfortable with this, you can begin to move him to his own room. The next step in this process would be to let him fall asleep in his own room, with you, and then you can move to your own bed after he falls asleep. This has worked for us.

Grooming: Haircuts

Here's what has worked for Alex. First we asked our parent network (there's that network again) for recommendations. We were pointed to a stylist who works for a children's salon here in NYC. Finding the right person, who is patient and ideally has experience cutting the hair of kids on the spectrum, is ideal. Next we arranged to come in before regular hours on the weekend (anyone that accommodates this is a keeper) before others arrive, which of course is a much calmer environment. The kid-focused salon also has the advantage of having TVs for distraction. I have also brought snacks and the iPad as well, though over time we've been able to phase this part out. Also beneficial for us has been giving a massage during the haircut.

I should also add, before we even go, I wash Alex's hair and discuss the upcoming haircut. We even have photos on the iPad of previous trips to get him ready for the transition. You can also video model the event or take photos for a social story. I've found that going on a consistent basis at consistent times helps fade out the agitation and anxiety over time.

~

Sensitivity to barbershop or salon odors: If this is the case, look for an old-fashioned barbershop that eschews smelly shampoos, or buy a home hair-cutting kit. Unscented products are often available, but you may have to buy them yourself and bring them in, or request them in advance.

~

Sensitivity to the sound of buzzing clippers or snapping scissors: Some people can tolerate one but not the other. There are also old-fashioned hand razors for cutting hair, but it's hard to find a barber who can wield one with precision. Call around! You might also try earplugs, or an iPod playing a favorite song through headphones. Your barber will happily work around headphones if it keeps the child in the chair. You might also choose to accept a longer hairstyle, if grooming is not a problem.

~

Sensory sensitivity in general. Try brushing the head and hair frequently with a medium-soft hairbrush. This may desensitize the area in time. You may be able to have your child sit in your lap during a haircut; a tight hug may calm him down. To begin, home haircuts may be your best bet.

Grooming: Toenail and Fingernail Clipping/Cleaning

Consistency is key here. Do on a regular basis; I have found most kids will gradually adapt to almost any task if its applied consistently, which is where parental willpower comes in.

~

With clipping, I model myself, and then do Alex. When first starting out, you can utilize an "if/then" process (if you do this, then you get that: food, swim etc). I've found this process useful in many cases to help accomplish an undesirable task, and have then been able to fade the "then" support over time.

~

Large, curved toenail clippers are easier to operate than small fingernail clippers and work fine for both fingernails and toenails. If possible, clip your child's nails while he is asleep to begin, but you eventually need to make this a regular routine event to overcome the anxiety.

~

Massage again: You can get improved compliance with a bit of a massage break between, say, each finger/toe. So clip, clean one finger, then massage shoulders, for instance.

Some Overall Useful Hygiene Tips

Most boys with autism do not learn what they need to know independently about hygiene and health, and this is an area that must be emphasized. Sometimes the lack of implementing has to do with the child having trouble remembering the steps or which routine to do when, and sometimes it is due to a lack of motor planning ability.

~

If there are problems with self-care, it is important to do a task analysis of where your boy is having trouble (i.e., never washes his hair) and then figure out why (i.e., he's forgetful; has a sensitive scalp; hates the feel/smell of the shampoo; hard to lift his arms that high up). Once you know what the problem is, you can find a solution.

~

Some boys like to wear the same thing over and over because of the feel of the fabric or the image on the shirt. This becomes unacceptable, as they get older. Tell him these clothes can be worn at home, in private (i.e., not when special guests are over). Find some comfortable replacements that are appropriate for his age for him to wear out of the house.

Good hygiene needs to be addressed in boys early on, and good habits developed and emphasized. Explain why it's important (social stories tailored to ability level). There are health reasons (we need to do this to stay healthy) and there are social reasons (we need to stay clean in order to make friends).

~

It's helpful to find a teen peer to go shopping with your son. You may think you know what is cool or "in," but a peer knows intuitively what the boys are wearing and what your son should wear. Looking like they fit in is really helpful, and encourages success in social situations with peers.

Siblings

It's important to remember that siblings of kids with autism have their own set of needs, which parents have to consider in raising a healthy family. Concerns include feelings of worry about their sibling with autism and jealousy of the attention required by their sibling. They may also have to help take care of and provide other levels of support in the community that their peers may not acknowledge, leading to possible resentment. Siblings can also feel guilt or anger over their duties and can feel ignored by parents due to the time siblings on the spectrum consume from parents.

This said, siblings who successfully adapt to the challenge are likely to be more loyal, supportive, and empathetic. More grown up. One way to help is to bring the sibling in on research or let them do part on their own, so they feel part of the team. Additionally, finding tasks or activities that both enjoy, such as watching a favorite show, swimming or certain video games, can create a special bond.

There are also sibling support groups in many schools and other run by various autism organizations around the country.

In addition to the challenges of having a sibling on the spectrum, there are also advantages:

- Growing up with a autism sibling means growing up with courage. Siblings learn what real challenges are and how to face them with strength.

188

- Siblings learn to mature at an early age; the need to support and stand up for their siblings means they often become wise beyond their years and tend to have greater compassion than peers.
- Whether it be communication challenges or other sensory and social issues, siblings learn to see the world in unique ways, which often makes them more creative and accepting than peers.

~

Siblings should have their own safe place, out of the way when you need to settle down or focus on your child with autism who may be melting down. After things calm down, return to your typical child and help him or her understand what occurred.

~

Let siblings be kids too! Don't expect sibs to become part-time parents. They can help out, sure, but allow them to aid in their own way, playing with or showing the child with autism how to play. Do not put a sib in the mode of babysitter.

When having a party, ask family members to help out. Organize a rotating team of adults, where each individual spends a half hour with the child, this allows parents and siblings to enjoy themselves, and the child doesn't have to be exposed to the chaos of the party.

~

Consider a sibling support group. If there aren't any in your area, there are books written for siblings of all ages.

Computer Time

Apps! Apps run on the iPhone, iTouch, and iPad providing a range of choices for your son. There are literally hundreds of autism related apps, just search for "autism" in the app store. Some favorites include: Proloquo2Go™, AutisMate, Avatalker (all are full-featured communication solutions), Is that Gluten Free?, Learn to Talk, iPrompts®, ABA Flash Cards, and iMean (which turns the entire screen into a large-button keyboard with text display).

~

Some children and adults with autism will learn more easily if the computer keyboard is placed close to the screen. This enables the individual to simultaneously see the keyboard and screen. Some individuals have difficulty remembering if they have to look up after they have hit a key on the keyboard.

> —*Temple Grandin, PhD, author of* Thinking in Pictures *and*
> The Way I See It; *www.autism.com/ind_teaching_tips.asp*

~

Temple Grandin often says that letting your child or teen spend too much time on the computer without a purpose is not a good idea. You do want to encourage computer skills to develop, as they may lead to job or career possibilities. To do that, Temple suggests finding a mentor to come over once a week to teach different computer applications and develop skill areas that could be helpful for future employment.

—Chantal Sicile-Kira

Finding Sitters/Home Help

As with most services, I have found the best sitters and helpers from other parents. You can also ask around at your son's school, camp, or play group. Many times some of the folks who work with the kids during the day are available to work at your home, either performing therapy or just supervising while you are out for a night of respite.

~

Check out your local colleges, which will usually post your sitter requests with the appropriate department, possibly in the special-needs education department. And join parent groups, organizations such as NAA and TACA, which will provide you with valuable parent connections.

~

The Medicaid waiver has two programs that help with home care. First is Community Rehabilitation, in which a worker comes into the home to work on specific skills, such as bathing, homework, etc. Hours and availability may vary by state (remember Medicaid is a state program) but generally you can get up to twelve hours per week broken out over three days. Oh, and did I mention it is free? The second program is called Respite and is also provided in the home. This is essentially babysitting, but another six to twelve hours per week (for free) is quite valuable. In many cases the programs have wait lists so check them out as early as possible. Additionally, if you have a worker in mind, you can send them to the waiver agency and the program itself then pays them direct. This could shorten the wait considerably.

Daily Anxiety

Child with anxiety? Recent research indicates that many on the spectrum have an imbalance in their Autonomic Nervous System (ANS), leading to sensory disorders. In these cases, children may have nausea, increased or racing heart rate, and dizziness. Migraines often are evident. Most of these troubles are the result of a stressed immune system. To alleviate this problem you can fix the immune system (which we'll leave to the docs/medical section) and balance the ANS.

There are many easy to implement strategies that can help balance your child's ANS:

- Cut electronic devices/TV off before bedtime, preferably an hour or two before; use this for reading time.
- Get enough sleep, eight hours a day and up.
- Exercise; target thirty minutes daily or at least every other day. Walking included.
- Learning. Taking on new information helps the brain exercise. Lumosity is a fun way, or some similar activity.
- Eliminate chemical exposure in foods, household, and beauty products (*suggestions below*).
- Positivity. Keeping things positive is key in so many facets.
- Listening to beautiful mellow music. If you have cable, check out the Soundscapes channel.
- Connect with nature. Best to combine this with the exercise above, but try and spend time each day in nature. Even if just taking a grounding walk barefoot in the backyard, along the beach, or in the park.

Eliminating Chemical Exposures

There are so many toxins used nowadays in everyday products it's a job in itself just to try and eliminate them. Really, it becomes a process of constant improvement. You'll learn to ferret out toxins over time, but the list below is a start.

- Remove all harmful chemical cleaning agents from your cleaning routine at home and at the office, and instead use cleaning products labeled "Level 1" by the EPA. Do not forget to include products for dishwashing and clothing detergent in your cleanup, and avoid toxic dry cleaning as much as possible.

- Improve your nutrition with a targeted vitamin supplementation program to include omega-3 essential fatty acids, sublingual methyl B-12, folinic acid, vitamin D3, zinc, and antioxidants.

- Eat organic, hormone-free food and avoid consuming fish or foods with MSG or food dyes.

- Drink organic green tea, filtered water, and antioxidant-rich organic juices while avoiding soda, carbonated beverages, and alcohol. With green tea, you want the powered type as most of the benefit of the drink is in ingesting the leaves.

- Use stevia, raw organic honey, and xylitol as sweeteners. Avoid any artificial sweeteners.

- Go for walks and get some sunshine daily.

- Cosmetics: Use aluminum-free natural deodorant, natural hennas to color hair, and avoid moisturizers or makeup with chemicals or parabens in them. Also avoid chemical dyes, perms, or other such hair treatments. Tom's is a great brand to try.

- Use only chemical-free cleaning products in your home, and avoid using pesticides or chemicals to treat your lawn.
- Watch the paper towels. Many commercial brands contain bleach as a whitener. Go with the green brands.

Chapter 10

Parting Suggestions

Nature does not hurry, yet everything is accomplished.

—*Lao Tzu*

Being Present

In this final chapter I'd like to share some suggestions and information I've learned over the years being Alex's dad. These are not Tips per se, but more akin to motivations to help along your journey. May they be as helpful to you as they have been to me.

~

Allowing Your Son to Be a Kid

Downtime is key, for both you and your child. I lay out many options for therapies and activities in this book, but do remember to take a breather now and then. A little R and R from each day is important. As part of this, let your child be involved in picking a relaxing activity or two each week. Give him the responsibility of coming up with something that interests him and involves a trip away from the work environment.

~

Grounding

Grounding is defined as having contact with the earth; think of walking barefoot in the grass or on the beach. Apparently when we have this kind of contact with the ground, we receive electrons, which have an antioxidant effect that helps our immune system function optimally leading to many beneficial results. There are some high-tech ways to accomplish this (just Google grounding) but I still prefer those outdoor walks. This might be a good option for those relaxing activities I mentioned above.

~

Surviving Tough Times

Everyone, especially autism parents, have gone through challenging times. And we all get through these times. Some, though, seem to come through easier and emerge stronger than before. The secret lies in staying present and maintaining a balanced mind-set. Below are some things to remember for the next challenge to get you to that balanced state.

- "Whether you think you can or can't—you're right." Mostly attributed to Henry Ford, many versions of this quote exist, but all have the same meaning. It's a problem if you think it's a problem. It all depends on your mind-set. If you allow your mind to see challenges as problems you are creating negative thoughts and emotions, which are not beneficial and have a way of leading to negative outcomes. If you view the challenge as something you can learn from, the problem dissipates.

- "It is what it is." Not sure where this exact version is from, but it traveled around in my Wall Street days. A version is attributed to Buddha though, and from here we learn that resistance leads to suffering. So suffering only occurs when we resist how things are. This does not imply non-action. In fact, the remainder of the Buddha version is to take action if you can change something. However, if you cannot change something then you can either obsess and create negativity, or accept what is and let go of the negative.

- "If you want things to change in your life, *you* have to change things in your life." There are other versions of this but all point toward the backwardness of thinking in regards to change we frequently have. If we want circumstances to change, things to be different than they are, then we need to change ourselves first. Take responsibility for change.

- Napoleon Hill in his well-known book, *Think and Grow Rich*, suggests to readers that they remove the word "failure" from their dictionaries. Not a bad idea. While it may seem that success is an overnight phenomena, all too often many "failures" precede success. Thomas Edison said, "I have not failed, I've just found 10,000 ways that do not work," in regards to his invention of the light bulb. If you are going to work to change things, you will have to fail from time to time, just take each setback as a learning opportunity.

- I mentioned earlier in this chapter about allowing your son to be a kid. In this vein, allow yourself to be happy and experience joy. Many people seem to be unable to allow the joy in and become addicted to their perceived problems. It becomes their identity. This, again, creates a negative mind, which attracts further negative thoughts and outcomes. So recognize this and permit yourself some joy from time to time to help break the pattern of suffering.

- Bad things don't happen to you, likewise, people don't "do things" to you. You are a victim only in your mind. It is you who create your own reality, experience and viewpoint. You have total responsibility for your mentality, how you label things. So put aside the idea of being a pawn or victim during challenging times and change your viewpoint.

- When things get tough, and they will again, remember, "Even when the sky is heavily overcast, the sun hasn't disappeared. It's still there on the other side of the clouds" (Eckhart Tolle). Just know that anything, including miracles, are possible and happen every day. I am sure you know of someone who overcame a tremendously challenging obstacle in life; if they can, you can. You just need to believe you can. Once you do, you will.

~

Being Happy

You know them, the people who when their name is mentioned are described as happy or positive. Are they just born that way? How do they do it? To be clear, I've typically had an optimistic outlook throughout life, but it has been tested. In my experience people who are always happy are that way regardless of challenges, they just don't fall into it, that is. So what do they do differently? How do they live their lives? Well . . .

- They are focused on the present but dream and plan for the future. If one is focused on the past, they will be depressed. If one is focused on the future, they will become anxious. Only by being present can happiness be achieved, as happiness is balance, the natural state. Just think of any object in the universe, all things seek balance, whether it be a star or a single atom.
- They don't bother trying to make others like them, because it does not matter if others like them. They like themselves first.

- They do things because they want to, not because they think they have to. So nobody can force them to do something, they act and do what they think is right regardless of outside views.

- When asked what "they do," happy folks do not answer with a job, title, or other ego driven response. They will say or describe specific things they are currently doing or working on, and these things usually involve the larger community. These things are also the things others seek to do when they "make it" or are "in a certain position." So happy folk dictate life, they are not dictated to by life.

- Happy folks love their friends but don't rely on them. They remain fully independent to avoid disappointment and thus do not harm the friendship.

- They are flexible and capable of moving or adapting to any environment or challenge. They may be content to follow a certain path and schedule for long periods of time, but are fully capable (without drama) of moving to another place, job, circumstance as opportunity/ challenge provide. There is no resistance. And yes, challenge = opportunity.

- They are not doctrinaire in their beliefs. Beliefs are constantly evolving and they don't judge how others live or their beliefs. They feel everyone is on their own path and that all require only that they follow the truth that satisfies them at present.

- They fear not death, as they know it is inevitable and only a transformation. After all, if all matter in the universe is truly energy, well energy cannot be destroyed, only transformed. It is only part of the process and must be necessary for it comes to all things.

- Finally, they do not try to change others, but seek to understand and inspire.

~

Right Before Bed

We all know the importance of sleep and I have discussed many aspects of it throughout the book. Often, the final thing or things done before bedtime dictates whether our sleep is successful or not. Here, I define a successful sleep as one that positively impacts energy and mood the next day. The following is a group of before bedtime rituals that many find useful for promoting a successful sleep.

- Read. Whether it be a book on autism, a fantasy novel, or some technical piece, nothing will induce a more successful sleep than reading just prior to bed. This ritual is easy to engage in, can be done with your child (and then on your own once they are down), and just gets you to that state of mind ready for relaxation. Combine with mellow soundscapes for a zen-like environment to wind up the day.

- Meditate. For thousands of years people have been using meditation to quiet the mind and make themselves receptive to a deeper realm. A practice that's been around for ages in multiple cultures must be on to something. Start with a brief 10-minute meditation. Look into a practice called Yoga Nidra. There are books and recordings available, many free. Often described as the "art of conscious relaxation," this guided practice is powerful and very easy to do and incorporate into your schedule. If you try anything on this list, try this.

- Keep a diary. Writing down or just listing what happened during the day allows a reflective release that is useful to creating a relaxed mind. Putting down on paper (electronic versions are okay, just do them a bit earlier, see below) symbolically allows your conscious to take a break and let the subconscious take over. Often upon waking solutions to vexations magically appear. Keep the diary nearby during the night, you may be compelled to jot down a sudden thought.

- Keep a list. Similarly, keeping a list of items you are working on and need to address the next day has that same reflective release mentioned above. As I've discussed multiple times, I keep a detailed spreadsheet or log of what I and Alex do each day. This is the perfect place to jot these lists/diary entries prior to bed. It also gives one a certain satisfaction of what was accomplished and subtly directs the mind to work on what needs to be done.

- Turn off. Yes, I mean TV, devices, email, and Facebook. All of these items are great helpers and time savers, but they also can easily be the cause of lost time and sleep. Nothing will keep you from a successful sleep like spending the final moments of the day watching or being stimulated by these visual imputs. Turn everything off an hour before bedtime.

- Speaking of bedtime, you need to have one. Sleep will not be successful if it's random. You need to have a time, or at least a range to begin with, so that your body recognizes what is expected of it. The same goes for your children of course. Ideally you would begin the rituals above at a similar time each night (yes, on the weekends too) and also wake up the following day at a similar time as well. We go down about the same time every night, but I will sleep in a bit more one day of the weekend to allow for a detox effect (going twelve plus hours without eating, mentioned elsewhere in this book).

~

Creating a No List

The ability to say no, also known as willpower, seems to be something that is in rare supply in our society nowadays.

Parting Suggestions

I have found the way to develop this power is exercise it. Create a No list of things that you will no longer accept as part of your life. Start with a single item, write it down in a visible place, and once you have developed it, add on. In this way the change is very subtle and manageable. Rushing into an extensive list (as often happens when folks diet) never works because you do not develop the discipline to maintain the gains. Nothing will come without discipline, but the great thing is, taking your time and working steadily at it is actually easier. Keep in mind the quote at the start of this chapter by Lao Tzu, "nature does not hurry, yet everything is accomplished." Here are some suggestions to get you started on your No list. Start with something that will be easy for you, and build that discipline for the tougher items that will come later.

- During dinner, no devices or TV. Play some calming music in the background.
- Do not sleep for less than eight hours a day. It's okay to start with six and work your way up.
- Do not go more than two days without some fitness activity. Eventually get this to daily.
- Avoid gossip and drama; you have enough on your plate.
- Do not use credit cards unless you pay them in full each month.
- Do not eat processed foods or "fast foods."

- Do not watch TV more than you read. Yes, this includes YouTube.
- Avoid listening to or watching negative programming.
- No more rushing!

Concluding Comments

Though this book is "short," I know there is a lot of information to consider and sample within. Just try and keep things as simple as possible when applying these tips. View the process as iterative: Some will work for you, and some will not. Take those that work for you and gradually work them into your daily routine.

It is my hope that you will discover even one tip in this compilation that will have a positive impact on your child's life, and your own. Write and tell us about it. We'd also love to hear any tips you may have. Send them to us, and they could make the next edition and land you a free copy of the book (signed, of course). You can send me a message at www.psychologytoday.com/experts/ken-siri. There, you can also read my updates on the *Psychology Today* blog.

Finally, remember you will need patience and optimism in this journey. Nobody can foretell the path your child will take and the spectrum of outcomes is broad. Take things step by step, stay present, and relish each day.

List of Contributors

Peggy Becker—pages 30–31
Mark L. Berger, CPA—pages 45–51
Joseph Campagna—pages 55–59
Stephanie Cave, MD—pages 39–40
Cathy Purple Cherry—pages 131–132, 142–143, 162–166, 178–179
Jennifer Clark—pages 128–129
Valorie Delp—pages 81–83
Karen Siff Exkorn—page 175
Mary Fetzer—page 101
Dr. Mark Frelich—pages 37, 88, 169–170
Ruby Gelman, DMD—pages 91, 92
Temple Grandin—pages 10–11, 67, 71–74, 79, 80–81, 121–122, 177, 189
Stanley Greenspan—pages 137–138
Laura Hynes—page 66
Markus Jarrow—pages 135, 136
Dr. Arthur Krigsman—pages 34, 35
Dr. Mary Jo Lang—pages 122–124
Maureen McDonnell, RN—pages 108–109
Lori McIlwain—pages 111–117
Lavinia Pereira—page 61
Kim Mack Rosenberg—pages 45–51
Chantal Sicile-Kira—page: 26, 67, 75, 151–152, 158–161, 169, 190
Michelle Solomon—page 61
Lauren Tobing-Puente, PhD—pages 20–21, 75–75
Tim Tucker—pages 101, 102, 104
Mitzi Waltz—pages 97–98

Resources

NATIONAL ORGANIZATIONS

ACT Today!
Autism Care & Treatment Today!
19019 Ventura Blvd. Suite 200
Tarzana, CA 91356
818-705-1625
Info@act-today.org
ACT Today! is a nonprofit organization whose mission is to provide funding and support to families that cannot afford the treatments their autistic children need to achieve their full potential.

Advancing Futures for Adults with Autism (AFAA)
917-475-5059
AFAA@autismspeaks.org
www.afaa-us.org
AFAA was created to inform adolescents and adults with autism about living options and new developments, and promote active community involvement from adults with autism.

Global Autism Collaboration
4182 Adams Avenue
San Diego, CA 92116
619-281-7165
www.autismwebsite.com/gac
The Global Autism Collaboration brings together the most experienced autism advocacy organizations in an effort dedicated to advancing autism research in the interest of all individuals living with autism today and their families.

The Autism Hope Alliance
752 Tamiami Trail
Port Charlotte, FL 33953
888-918-1118
info@autismhopealliance.org
Dedicated to the recovery of children and adults from autism, the Autism Hope Alliance ignites hope for families facing the diagnosis through education

and funding to promote progress in the present moment.

AutismOne
1816 W. Houston Avenue
Fullerton, CA 92833
714-680-0792
earranga@autismone.org
www.autismone.org
AutismOne is a nonprofit, charity organization educating more than 100,000 families every year about prevention, recovery, safety, and change.

Autism Research Institute
4182 Adams Avenue
San Diego, CA 92116
619-281-7165
Media Contact: Matt Kabler
matt@autism.com
www.autism.com
ARI is devoted to conducting research and to disseminating the results of research on the triggers of autism and on methods of diagnosing and treating autism.

Autism Science Digest
1816 W. Houston Ave.

Fullerton, CA 92833
714-680-0792
Contact: Teri Arranga, Editor in Chief
tarranga@autismone.org
www.autismsciencedigest.com
Autism Science Digest is the place for doctors, researchers, and expert mothers and fathers to get together to talk about research, treatment, and recovery. *Autism Science Digest* is the first Autism Approved™ publication of the global autism community. Dedicated to respecting the intelligence of parents, *Autism Science Digest* continues the philosophy of founding organization, AutismOne, featuring up-to-date biomedical information written for new and seasoned readers from clinicians and researchers you trust.

Autism Society
4340 East-West Hwy, Suite 350
Bethesda, MD 20814
www.autism-society.org
301-657-0881,
1-800-3AUTISM x 150

info@autism-society.org

The Autism Society exists to improve the lives of all affected by autism by increasing public awareness about the day-to-day issues faced by people on the spectrum, advocating for appropriate services for individuals across the lifespan, and providing the latest information regarding treatment, education, research, and advocacy.

Autism Speaks

2 Park Avenue, 11th Floor
New York, NY 10016
212-252-8584
contactus@autismspeaks.org
www.autismspeaks.org
Autism Speaks is dedicated to funding autism research, disseminating information, and providing a voice for autistic people's needs.

The Canary Party

admin@canaryparty.org
Toll Free 855-711-5282
www.canaryparty.org
650-471-8897

The Canary Party is a movement created to stand up for the victims of medical injury, environmental toxins, and industrial foods by restoring balance to our free and civil society and empowering consumers to make health and nutrition decisions that promote wellness.

Generation Rescue

19528 Ventura Blvd. #117
Tarzana, CA 91356
1-877-98-AUTISM
www.generationrescue.org
Generation Rescue is Jenny McCarthy's autism organization dedicated to informing and assisting families touched by autism; it provides programs and services for personalized support, and Generation Rescue volunteers are researching causes and treatment for autism.

Helping Hand

1330 W. Schatz Lane
Nixa, MO 65714
877-NAA-AUTISM
(877-622-2884)

naa@nationalautism.org
www.nationalautismassociation.
org/helpinghand.php
Helping Hand is a program
from the National Autism
Association that provides
financial assistance for autism
families.

**Kids Enjoy Exercise
Now (KEEN)**
1301 K Street, NW
Suite 600, East Tower
Washington, DC 20005
866-903-KEEN (5336) main
866-597-KEEN (5336) fax
info@keenusa.org
KEEN is a national, nonprofit
volunteer-led organization
that provides one-to-one
recreational opportunities
for children and young
adults with developmental
and physical disabilities at
no cost to their families and
caregivers. KEEN's mission
is to foster the self-esteem,
confidence, skills and talents
of its athletes through
non-competitive activities,
allowing young people facing

even the most significant
challenges to meet their
individual goals.

**National Autism
Association**
1330 W. Schatz Lane
Nixa, MO 65714
877-622-2884
naa@nationalautism.org
www.nationalautism.org
NAA raises funds for autism
research and support and also
provides programs, such as
Helping Hand, Family First,
and FOUND, designed to
aid specific needs for families
dealing with autism.

National Autism Center
41 Pacella Park Drive
Randolph, Massachusetts 02368
Phone: 877-313-3833
Fax: 781-440-0401
Email: info@
nationalautismcenter.org
www.nationalautismcenter.org
The National Autism Center
is a nonprofit organization
dedicated to serving children
and adolescents with

Resources

Autism Spectrum Disorders
(ASD) by providing reliable
information, promoting
best practices, and offering
comprehensive resources for
families, practitioners, and
communities.

Organization for Autism Research

2000 North 14th Street
Suite 710
Arlington, VA 22201
Tel: 703-243-9710
www.researchautism.org
The Organization for Autism
Research (OAR) was created
in December 2001—the
product of the shared vision
and unique life experiences of
OAR's seven founders. Led by
these parents and grandparents
of children and adults on the
autism spectrum, OAR set
out to use applied science to
answer questions that parents,
families, individuals with
autism, teachers and caregivers
confront daily. No other autism
organization has this singular
focus.

SafeMinds

16033 Bolsa Chica St. #104-142
Huntington Beach, CA 92649
404-934-0777
www.safeminds.org
SafeMinds is an organization
dedicated to research and
awareness of mercury's
involvement in such
neurological disorders as
autism, attention deficit
disorder, and more.

Talk About Curing Autism (TACA)

3070 Bristol Street, Suite 340
Costa Mesa CA 92626
949-640-4401
www.tacanow.org
TACA provides medical, diet,
and educational information
geared toward autistic children,
and the organization also
has support, resources, and
community events.

U.S. Autism and Asperger Association

P.O. Box 532
Draper, UT 84020-0532
888-9AUTISM, 801-649-5752

information@usautism.org
www.usautism.org
USAAA provides support, education, and resources for autistic individuals and those with Asperger's Syndrome.

Unlocking Autism
P.O. Box 208
Tyrone, GA 30290
866-366-3361
www.unlockingautism.org
Unlocking Autism was created to find information about autism and disseminate that information to families with autistic children; the organization also raises funds for research and awareness.

ONLINE ORGANIZATIONS

Age of Autism
www.ageofautism.com
Age of Autism is an online blog with daily news in the latest autism research, updates, and community happenings.

Foundation for Autism Information & Research, Inc.
1300 Jefferson Rd.
Hoffman Estates, IL 60169
info@autismmedia.org
F.A.I.R. Autism Media is a non-profit foundation creating original, up-to-date and comprehensive educational media (video documentaries) to inform the medical community and the public about the latest advances in research and biomedical & behavioral therapies for autism spectrum disorders.

Schafer Autism Report
9629 Old Placerville Road
Sacramento, CA 95827
edit@doitnow.com
www.sarnet.org
Schafer Autism Report is a publication to inform the public about autism-related issues; it can be found online.

Suggested Reading

Adams, Christina, *A Real Boy*. Berkley Books, 2005.

Bailey, Sally, *Wings to Fly: Bringing Theatre Arts to Students with Special Needs* (Woodbine House, 1993) and *Barrier-Free Drama*

Barbera, Mary Lynch, and Tracy Rasmussen. *The Verbal Behavior Approach: How to Teach Children with Autism and Related Disorders.* Jessica Kingsley Publishers, 2007.

Bluestone, Judith. *The Fabric of Autism: Weaving the Threads into a Cogent Theory.* The HANDLE Institute, 2004.

Bock, Kenneth, and Cameron Stauth. *Healing the New Childhood Epidemics: Autism, ADHD, Asthma, and Allergies: The Groundbreaking Program for the 4-A Disorders.* Ballantine Books, 2008.

Buckley, Julie A. *Healing Our Autistic Children: A Medical Plan.* Palgrave Macmillan 2010.

Casanova, Manuel F. *Brain, Behavior and Evolution* magazines, *Recent Developments in Autism Research* (Nova Biomedical Books, 2005), *Asperger's Disorder* (Medical Psychiatry Series) [Informa Healthcare, 2008], *Neocortical Modularity And The Cell Minicolumn* (Nova Biomedical Books, 2005)

Chauhan, Abha, Ved Chauhan, and Ted Brown, editors. *Autism: Oxidative Stress, Inflammation, and Immune Abnormalities.* CRC Press, 2009.

Chinitz, Judith Hope, *We Band of Mothers: Autism, My Son, and the Specific Carbohydrate Diet* (Autism Research Institute, 2007)

Davis, Dorinne S., *Every Day A Miracle: Success Stories through Sound Therapy*. Kalco Publishing LLC (October 6, 2004)

Davis, Dorinne. *Sound Bodies through Sound Therapy.* Kalco Publishing LLC, 2004.

Delaine, Susan K. *The Autism Cookbook: 101 Gluten-Free and Dairy-Free Recipes.* Skyhorse Publishing, 2010.

Fine, Aubrey, and Nya M. Fine, editors. *Therapeutic Recreation for Exceptional Children : Let Me In, I Want to Play*. Delta Society, 1996.

Fine and Eisen. *Afternoons with Puppy*. Purdue University Press 2008.

Fine, Aubrey. *The Handbook on Animal Assisted Therapy: Theoretical Foundations and Guidelines for Practice*. Academic Press, 1999.

Gabriels, R. "Art therapy with children who have autism and their families." *Handbook of art therapy*. Ed. C. Malchiodi. Guilford Press, 2003.

Grandin, Temple, *The Way I See It*. Future Horizons, 2011.

Goldberg, Michael J., with Elyse Goldberg. *The Myth of Autism: How a Misunderstood Epidemic Is Destroying Our Children*. Skyhorse Publishing, 2011.

Gottschall, Elaine G. *Breaking the Vicious Cycle: Intestinal Health Through Diet*. Kirkton Press, 1994.

Gillman, Priscilla, *The Anti-Romantic Child*. Harper Perennial.

Grandin, Temple and Catherine Johnson. *Animals in Translation Using the Mysteries of Autism to Decode Animal Behavior*. Houghton Mifflin Harcourt, 2005.

Greenspan, Stabley and Wieder, Serena. *Engaging Autism: Using the Floortime Approach to Help Children Relate, Communicate, and Think*. Da Capo Press, 2006.

Greenspan, Stanley, with Jacob Greenspan. *Overcoming ADHD: Helping Your Child Become Calm, Engaged, and Focused—Without a Pill*. Da Capo Lifelong Books, 2009.

Grinspoon, Lester, *Marihuana Reconsidered* (Harvard University press 1971, 1977, and American archives press classic edition, 1994) and *Marijuana, the Forbidden Medicine* (Yale University press, 1993, 1997)

Heflin, Juane, *Spectrum Disorders: Effective Instructional Practices* (Prentice Hall, 2006)

Suggested Reading

Henley, D. R. *Exceptional children, exceptional art: Teaching art to special needs.* Worcester, MA: Davis Publications, 1992.

Herskowitz, Valerie. *Autism & Computers: Maximizing Independence Through Technology.* AuthorHouse, 2009.

Heflin, L. Juane. *Students with Autism Spectrum Disorders: Effective Instructional Practices,* Prentice Hall, 2007.

Hogenboom, Marga. *Living with Genetic Syndromes Associated with Intellectual Disability.* Jessica Kingsley Publishers, 2001.

Jepson, Bryan Jepson. *Changing the Course of Autism: A Scientific Approach for Parents and Physicians.* Sentient Publications, 2007.

Kaufman, Barry Neil. *Son Rise: The Miracle Continues.* H J Kramer, 1994.

Kawar, Frick and Frick. *Astronaut Training: A Sound Activated Vestibular-Visual Protocol for Moving, Looking & Listening.* Vital Sounds LLC, 2006.

Kirby, David. *Evidence of Harm: Mercury in Vaccines and the Autism Epidemic: A Medical Controversy.* St. Martin's Press, 2005.

Kranowitz, Carol Stock, *The Out-of-Sync Child.* Perigee, 2005.

Lansky, Amy L. *Impossible Cure: The Promise of Homeopathy.* R.L. Ranch Press, 2003.

Lewis, Lisa. *Special Diets For Special Kids I & II.* Future Horizons, 2001.

Levinson, B. M. *Pet-oriented Child Psychotherapy.* Springfield, IL: Charles C. Thomas. 1969.

Lyons, Tony. *1,001 Tips for the Parents of Autistic Girls: Everything You Need to Know About Diagnosis, Doctors, Schools, Taxes, Vacations, Babysitters, Treatment, Food, and More.* Skyhorse Publishing, 2010.

Marohn, Stephanie. *The Natural Medicine Guide to Autism.* Hampton Roads Pub Co, 2002.

Martin, Nicole. *Art as an Early Intervention Tool for Children with Autism.* Jessica Kingsley Publishers, 2009.

Matthews, Julie. *Nourishing Hope for Autism: Nutrition Intervention for Healing Our Children, 3rd ed.* Healthful Living Media, 2008.

217

Maurice, Catherine. *Let Me Hear Your Voice: A Family's Triumph over Autism*. Ballantine Books, 1994.

McCandless, Jaquelyn. *Children with Starving Brains: A Medical Treatment Guide for Autism Spectrum Disorder, 4th ed.* Bramble Books, 2009.

McCarthy, Jenny and Jerry Kartzinel. *Healing and Preventing Autism: A Complete Guide*. Penguin, 2009.

McCarthy, Jenny. *Louder Than Words: A Mother's Journey in Healing Autism*. Penguin, 2007.

McCarthy, Jenny. *Mother Warriors*. Penguin, 2008.

Mehl-Madrona, Lewis, *Coyote Medicine* (Touchstone, 1998), *Coyote Healing* (Bear & Company, 2003) *Coyote Wisdom* (Bear & Company, 2005) *Narrative Medicine* (Bear & Company, 2007) and *Healing the Mind through the Power of Story: The Promise of Narrative Psychiatry* (Bear & Company (June 15, 2010)).

Noble, J. "Art as an instrument for creating social reciprocity: Social skills group for children with autism." *Group process made visible: Group art therapy*. Ed. S. Riley. Brunner-Routledge, 2001.

Pereira, Lavinia, and Solomon Michelle, *First Sound Series* by Trafford Publishing

Prizant, Barry, Amy Wetherby, Emily Rubin, Amy Laurent and P. Rydell. *The SCERTS Model: A Comprehensive Educational Approach for Children with Autism Spectrum Disorders*. Baltimore, MD: Paul H. Brookes Publishing, 2006.

Rimland, Bernard. *Infantile Autism: The Syndrome and Its Implication for a Neural Theory of Behavior*. Prentice Hall, 1964.

Rimland, Bernard, Jon Pangborn, Sidney Baker. *Autism: Effective Biomedical Treatments (Have We Done Everything We Can For This Child? Individuality In An Epidemic)*. Autism Research Institute, 2005.

Rimland, Bernard, Jon Pangborn, Sidney Baker. *2007 Supplement - Autism: Effective Biomedical Treatments (Have We Done Everything*

We Can for This Child? Individuality In An Epidemic). Autism Research Institute, 2007.

Robbins, Jim. *A Symphony in the Brain: The Evolution of the New Brain Wave Biofeedback*. Grove Press, 2008.

Rogers, Sally J. and Geraldine Dawson. *Early Start Denver Model For Young Children With Autism: Promoting Language, Learning, And Engagement*. Guilford Press, 2009.

Seroussi, Karyn. *Unraveling the Mystery of Autism and Pervasive Developmental Disorders*. Simon & Schuster, 2000.

Seroussi, Karyn and Lisa Lewis. *The Encyclopedia of Dietary Interventions for the Treatment of Autism and Related Disorders*. Sarpsborg Press, 2008.

Sicile-Kira, Chantal. *Autism Spectrum Disorders: The Complete Guide to Understanding Autism, Asperger's Syndrome, Pervasive Developmental Disorder, and Other ASDs*. Penguin, 2004.

Sicile-Kira, Chantal. *Adolescents on the Autism Spectrum: A Parent's Guide to the Cognitive, Social, Physical, and Transition Needs of Teenagers with Autism Spectrum Disorders*. Penguin, 2006.

Sicile-Kira, Chantal. *Autism Life Skills: From Communication and Safety to Self-Esteem and More — 10 Essential Abilities Every Child Needs and Deserves to Learn*. Penguin, 2008.

Sicile-Kira, Chantal, *A Full Life with Autism*. Palgrave MacMillan, 2012.

Silva, Louisa. *Helping your Child with Autism: A Home Program from Chinese Medicine*. Guan Yin Press, 2010.

Silver, R. A. *Developing cognitive and creative skills through art: Programs for children with communication disorders or learning disabilities* (3rd ed. revised). New York: Albin Press 1989.

Siri, Kenneth, *1001 Tips for Parents of Autistic Boys*. Skyhorse Publishing, 2010.

Stagliano, Kim. *All I Can Handle: I'm No Mother Teresa: A Life Raising Three Daughters with Autism*. Skyhorse Publishing, 2010.

Theoharides, Theoharis C., *Pharmacology* (Essentials of Basic Science) (Little Brown and Company, 1992) *Essentials of Pharmacology* (Essentials of Basic Science) (Lippincott Williams & Wilkins, 1996)

Wiseman, Nancy D. *The First Year: Autism Spectrum Disorders: An Essential Guide for the Newly Diagnosed Child.* Da Capo Lifelong Books, 2009.

Wolfberg, Pamela J. *Play and Imagination in Children with Autism, 2nd ed.* Autism Asperger Publishing Company, 2009.

Woodward, Bob and Marga Hogenboom. *Autism: A Holistic Approach.* Floris Books, 2001.

Yasko, Amy. *Autism: Pathways to Recovery.* Neurological Research Institute, 2009.

Yasko, Amy. *Genetic Bypass: Using Nutrition to Bypass Genetic Mutations.* Neurological Research Institute, 2005.

Acknowledgements

I would like to thank my Skyhorse Publishing editors
Joseph Sverchek and Maxim Brown, without whom I could
not have completed this project. I would also like to thank
Chantal Sicile-Kira, Kim Mack Rosenberg, Mark Berger,
Joseph Campagna, Temple Grandin, Cathy Purple Cherry,
and Lori McIlwain, all of whom provided significant
contributions and filled in gaps in my experience and
knowledge to help make this book more comprehensive.

A special thanks to my friends who have joined Alex
and I on this journey, the Calle Ocho crew including,
Amanda, Alison, Tony, Kim, Peggy, Dara & Mark, Loren, Joe
& Jennifer, Alpin, Joey, Aaron, Lesly, and Jennifer C. Looking
forward to the next mojito!

And to my son Alex, who has transformed my life in
so many positive ways, taught me presence, and inspires me
daily.

Cheers,
Ken

Index

Index

Index

Index

Index

Index

Index

Index